THE DR. NOWZARADAN 1200-CALORIE DIET PLAN

Enjoy Healthy Eating and Lose Weight with Dr. Nowzaradan's 90-Day Meal Plan of Delicious, Low-Carb, High-Protein Recipes to Support Your Journey

Eva Mcgee

© Copyright 2024 by Eva Mcgee - All rights reserved.

The following book is provided below with the aim of delivering information that is as precise and dependable as possible. However, purchasing this book implies an acknowledgment that both the publisher and the author are not experts in the discussed topics, and any recommendations or suggestions contained herein are solely for entertainment purposes. It is advised that professionals be consulted as needed before acting on any endorsed actions.

This statement is considered fair and valid by both the American Bar Association and the Committee of Publishers Association, and it holds legal binding throughout the United States.

Moreover, any transmission, duplication, or reproduction of this work, including specific information, will be deemed an illegal act, regardless of whether it is done electronically or in print. This includes creating secondary or tertiary copies of the work or recorded copies, which are only allowed with the express written consent from the Publisher. All additional rights are reserved.

The information in the following pages is generally considered to be a truthful and accurate account of facts. As such, any negligence, use, or misuse of the information by the reader will result in actions falling solely under their responsibility. There are no scenarios in which the publisher or the original author can be held liable for any difficulties or damages that may occur after undertaking the information described herein.

Additionally, the information in the following pages is intended solely for informational purposes and should be considered as such. As fitting its nature, it is presented without assurance regarding its prolonged validity or interim quality. Mention of trademarks is done without written consent and should not be construed as an endorsement from the trademark holder.

TABLE OF CONTENTS

INTRODUCTION 7
- 1. Starting Your Weight Loss Journey 7
- 2. Decoding the 1200-Calorie Mystery 9

CHAPTER 1: UNDERSTANDING THE DR. NOW APPROACH 11
- 1. The Core Philosophy 11
- 2. The Science Behind the Diet 12
- 3. Setting Realistic Goals 14
- 4. Customizing the Plan to Individual Needs 15
- 5. Psychological Aspects of Dieting 16

CHAPTER 2: THE POWER OF NUTRITION 19
- 1. Health Benefits of Eating Right 19
- 2. Common Nutritional Pitfalls 20
- 3. Building a Balanced Diet 22
- 4. Essential Nutrients and Where to Find Them 23
- 5. Anti-Inflammatory Foods for Longevity 25

CHAPTER 3: THE 90-DAY MEAL PLAN 27
- 1. Introduction to the Meal Plan 27

CHAPTER 4: BREAKFAST OPTIONS 29
- 1. Quick and Easy Recipes 29
- 2. Balanced Breakfast Meals 32
- 3. Prep-Ahead Ideas 35

CHAPTER 5: LUNCH SOLUTIONS 39
- 1. Nutrient-Dense Salads 39
- 2. Hearty Soups and Stews 43
- 3. Portable Lunches 46

CHAPTER 6: DINNER DELIGHTS 51
- 1. Lean Proteins 51
- 2. Vegetable-Centric Meals 54
- 3. Comfort Foods Made Healthy 58

CHAPTER 7: DESSERTS AND TREATS 63
    1. Low-Calorie Desserts 63
    2. Healthy Baking 64
    3. Indulgent Yet Guilt-Free 66

CHAPTER 8: STAYING MOTIVATED 67
    1. Maintaining Momentum 67
    2. Overcoming Challenges 68
    3. Long-Term Success 70
    4. Celebrating Milestones 71
    Measurement Conversion Table 73

INTRODUCTION

1. STARTING YOUR WEIGHT LOSS JOURNEY

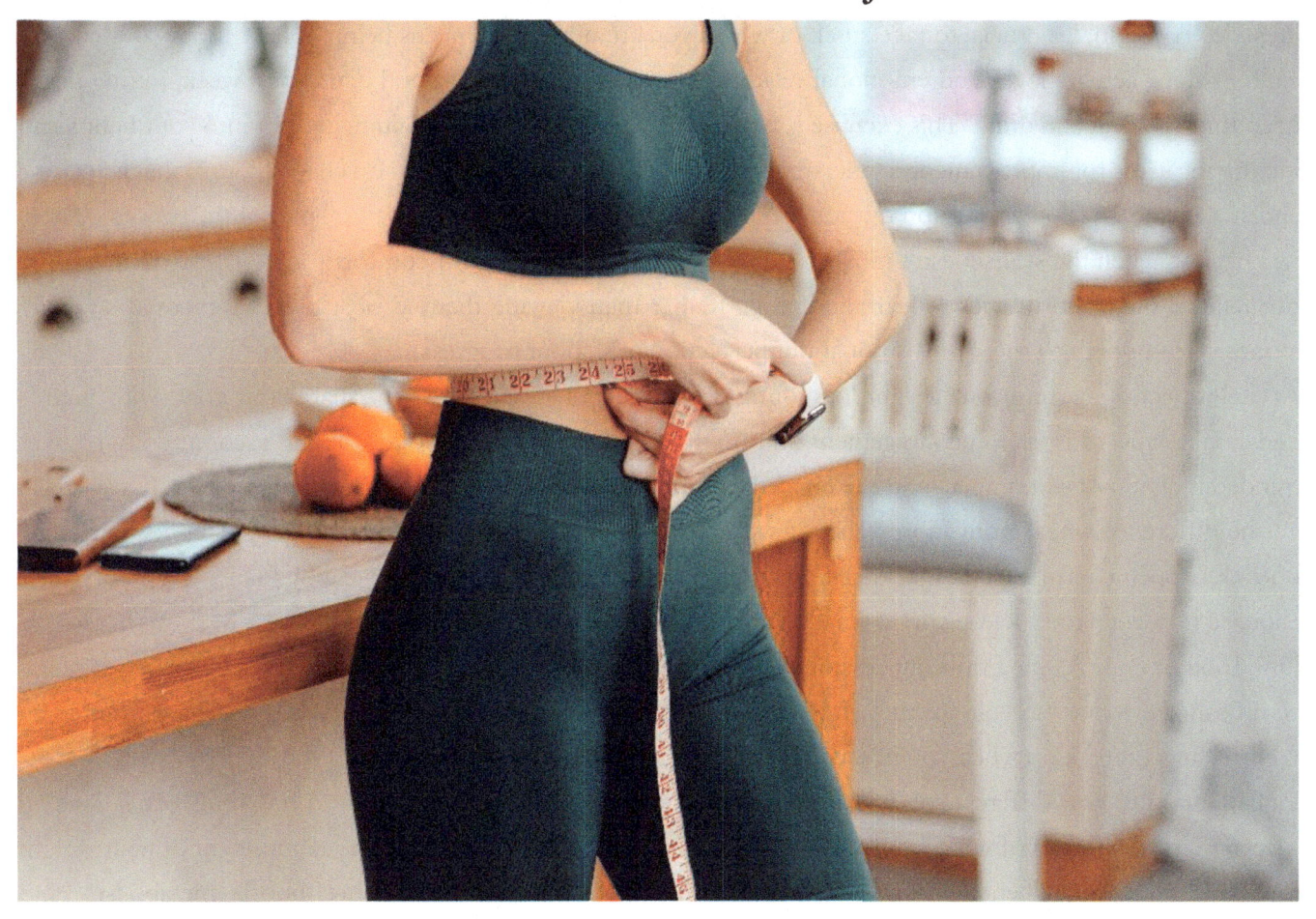

In the hustle and bustle of everyday life, embarking on a weight loss journey can feel daunting. Yet, the decision to pursue a healthier lifestyle is a profound commitment to yourself and your well-being. As you stand at the crossroads of change, it's essential to embrace this journey with optimism, determination, and an open heart.

The first step is acknowledging why you're here. For many, the path to weight loss is paved with a desire to improve health, boost energy, and reclaim control over one's body. Perhaps you've felt the frustration of diets that promised miracles but delivered little more than fleeting results. Or maybe you're tired of feeling trapped in a cycle of yo-yo dieting and self-doubt. Whatever your motivation, know that you are not alone.

Embarking on this journey is as much about the mind as it is about the body. It requires a shift in mindset, from seeing food as an adversary to embracing it as nourishment. Understanding the power of nutrition and how it impacts your body is crucial. Dr. Nowzaradan's approach provides a framework that is not just about counting calories but about making informed choices that fuel your body and support your health.

It's important to start by setting realistic and achievable goals. Weight loss is not a sprint; it's a marathon that requires patience and persistence. Begin by asking yourself what you want to achieve and why. Is it to feel more comfortable in your skin, to improve your health markers, or to set a positive example for your family? Whatever your reasons, write them down. Keep them in a place where you can see them daily, reminding yourself of your 'why' when the going gets tough. One of the most significant challenges in any weight loss journey is navigating the sea of information. Diet trends come and go, each claiming to hold the key to quick and easy weight loss.

It's easy to feel overwhelmed by conflicting advice and wonder which path is right for you. The truth is, there is no one-size-fits-all solution. The best approach is one that fits seamlessly into your life and meets your unique needs. That's where this plan comes in, offering a structured yet flexible guide that you can adapt to suit your lifestyle. To begin, it's crucial to take stock of where you are now. This means being honest about your current eating habits, activity level, and emotional relationship with food. Keep a food diary for a week, jotting down everything you eat and drink. This exercise is not about judgment but about gaining insight into your habits and identifying areas for improvement. Understanding your starting point will help you chart a course that is realistic and sustainable. As you embark on this journey, remember that setbacks are a natural part of the process. There will be days when the scale doesn't move, or you find yourself reaching for comfort foods. These moments are not failures but opportunities to learn and grow. Rather than viewing them as obstacles, see them as stepping stones on your path to success. It's not about perfection; it's about progress.

A vital aspect of starting your weight loss journey is building a support system. Share your goals with friends and family who can offer encouragement and hold you accountable. Consider joining a community of like-minded individuals who understand the challenges and triumphs you face. Having people to lean on can make all the difference when motivation wanes. As you delve into the 90-day meal plan, keep in mind that change doesn't happen overnight. Allow yourself grace and patience as you adapt to new eating habits and incorporate exercise into your routine. Celebrate small victories along the way, whether it's choosing a healthy snack over junk food or completing a workout session. These accomplishments, no matter how minor they may seem, are significant milestones in your journey. It's also essential to listen to your body and honor its signals. Eat when you're hungry, and stop when you're satisfied.

Pay attention to how different foods make you feel, both physically and emotionally. Over time, you'll develop a deeper understanding of what your body needs to thrive. Hydration is another key component of your weight loss journey. Drinking enough water throughout the day helps regulate appetite, boosts metabolism, and supports overall health. Aim to replace sugary beverages with water or herbal teas, and notice how much better you feel as a result. In addition to nutrition, incorporating regular physical activity is vital. Find activities that you enjoy, whether it's walking, dancing, swimming, or yoga. Exercise should not be a punishment but a celebration of what your body can do. Start small, gradually increasing the intensity and duration as your fitness improves.

Mindfulness can be a powerful tool in your weight loss journey. Practice being present during meals, savoring each bite, and appreciating the flavors and textures. Mindful eating helps prevent overeating and fosters a healthier relationship with food. Additionally, mindfulness techniques such as meditation and deep breathing can reduce stress, which often triggers emotional eating. As you embark on this transformative journey, keep your focus on long-term success. This is not a quick fix but a lifestyle change that requires commitment and dedication. Be kind to yourself, recognizing that progress takes time. The habits you form now will lay the foundation for a healthier future.

In closing, starting your weight loss journey is an empowering step towards a healthier, happier you. Embrace the process with an open mind and a willingness to learn. Trust in your ability to make positive changes, and believe in the possibility of success. Remember, you are not just losing weight; you are gaining a new perspective on life and a renewed sense of vitality. Your journey has just begun, and the possibilities are endless. Stay committed, stay focused, and most importantly, stay true to yourself. As you progress through this book, you'll discover tools, tips, and recipes to support you every step of the way. Here's to the beginning of a healthier you, filled with hope, resilience, and determination. Let's embark on this journey together, one step at a time.

2. DECODING THE 1200-CALORIE MYSTERY

The 1200-calorie diet plan often finds itself in the spotlight, a seemingly magical number for weight loss that has captured the interest of many. Yet, what makes this specific number so compelling, and why has it become a cornerstone in weight management strategies? To understand its appeal and effectiveness, it's essential to delve into the science and rationale behind it. This exploration reveals not just a caloric value but a thoughtful approach to balancing nutrition and achieving sustainable results.

At its core, the 1200-calorie diet is designed to create a calorie deficit, a fundamental principle of weight loss. When you consume fewer calories than your body expends, your body taps into stored fat for energy, leading to weight loss. The figure of 1200 calories is often suggested because it is low enough to encourage weight loss in most individuals but high enough to provide adequate nutrition for daily functioning. It's a balance between efficiency and safety, designed to support weight loss while minimizing the risk of nutritional deficiencies.

For many, 1200 calories represent a significant reduction in daily intake. It's a change that requires careful planning and mindful eating. This is where the real work begins: crafting meals that are not only calorie-conscious but also rich in nutrients. The goal is to maximize nutritional value while keeping calories low. This approach emphasizes whole, unprocessed foods that provide the vitamins, minerals, and other nutrients your body needs to function optimally. Imagine your daily calorie allotment as a budget. You want to spend it wisely, choosing foods that offer the greatest nutritional bang for your buck. This often means focusing on foods that are high in fiber and protein, as these nutrients help keep you feeling full and satisfied. Vegetables, lean proteins, whole grains, and healthy fats become staples in this diet, providing the sustenance you need without tipping the calorie scale. The concept of the 1200-calorie diet can also serve as a framework for learning about portion control and mindful eating. When every calorie counts, you become more aware of what you're eating and why. This heightened awareness can lead to more intentional food choices and a deeper understanding of how different foods affect your body and energy levels. It's an educational process as much as it is a dietary strategy, teaching you to listen to your body's hunger cues and make informed decisions about what to eat.

However, it's crucial to recognize that the 1200-calorie diet isn't a one-size-fits-all solution. Individual needs vary based on factors such as age, gender, activity level, and overall health. What works for one person may not be suitable for another. Therefore, it's important to approach this diet with flexibility, making adjustments as needed to fit your personal needs and goals. Consulting with a healthcare professional or nutritionist can provide personalized guidance and ensure that the diet is appropriate for your situation.

The effectiveness of the 1200-calorie diet is not just in its ability to promote weight loss but also in how it encourages sustainable lifestyle changes. It requires planning and commitment, habits that can lead to long-term success beyond the diet itself. The skills you develop—meal planning, portion control, mindful eating—are valuable tools that support lasting weight management. One of the challenges of a reduced-calorie diet is ensuring you still enjoy your meals. Eating should be a pleasurable experience, not a chore. This is where creativity in the kitchen comes into play. Experimenting with flavors, trying new recipes, and discovering healthy alternatives can keep your meals exciting and enjoyable. The key is to make the diet work for you, finding ways to satisfy your palate while staying within your calorie goals.

It's also important to consider the psychological aspects of dieting. The 1200-calorie diet, like any dietary change, requires mental resilience and a positive mindset. It's about shifting your perspective from deprivation to empowerment. Instead of focusing on what you can't have, celebrate the delicious and nutritious foods you can enjoy. This mindset fosters a healthier relationship with food, where you view it as nourishment rather than an enemy. Support can play a crucial role in the success of a 1200-calorie diet. Whether it's a friend, family member, or support group, having someone to share the journey with can provide encouragement and accountability. Sharing tips, recipes, and progress can make the experience more rewarding and less isolating. Community support can also offer motivation during challenging times, reminding you of your goals and the reasons you started this journey. While the 1200-calorie diet can be an effective tool for weight loss, it's important to focus on the bigger picture of health and well-being. True success is not just about reaching a certain weight but also about feeling good in your body, having energy, and enjoying life. The 1200-calorie framework is a stepping stone toward these broader goals, providing a structure that supports a healthy lifestyle.

In conclusion, the 1200-calorie diet is more than just a number. It's a thoughtful approach to weight management that emphasizes nutrition, mindfulness, and sustainability. By focusing on nutrient-dense foods and embracing healthy habits, you can achieve your weight loss goals while nurturing your body and mind. This journey is about more than just losing weight; it's about gaining health, confidence, and a new perspective on living well.

CHAPTER 1: UNDERSTANDING THE DR. NOW APPROACH
1. THE CORE PHILOSOPHY

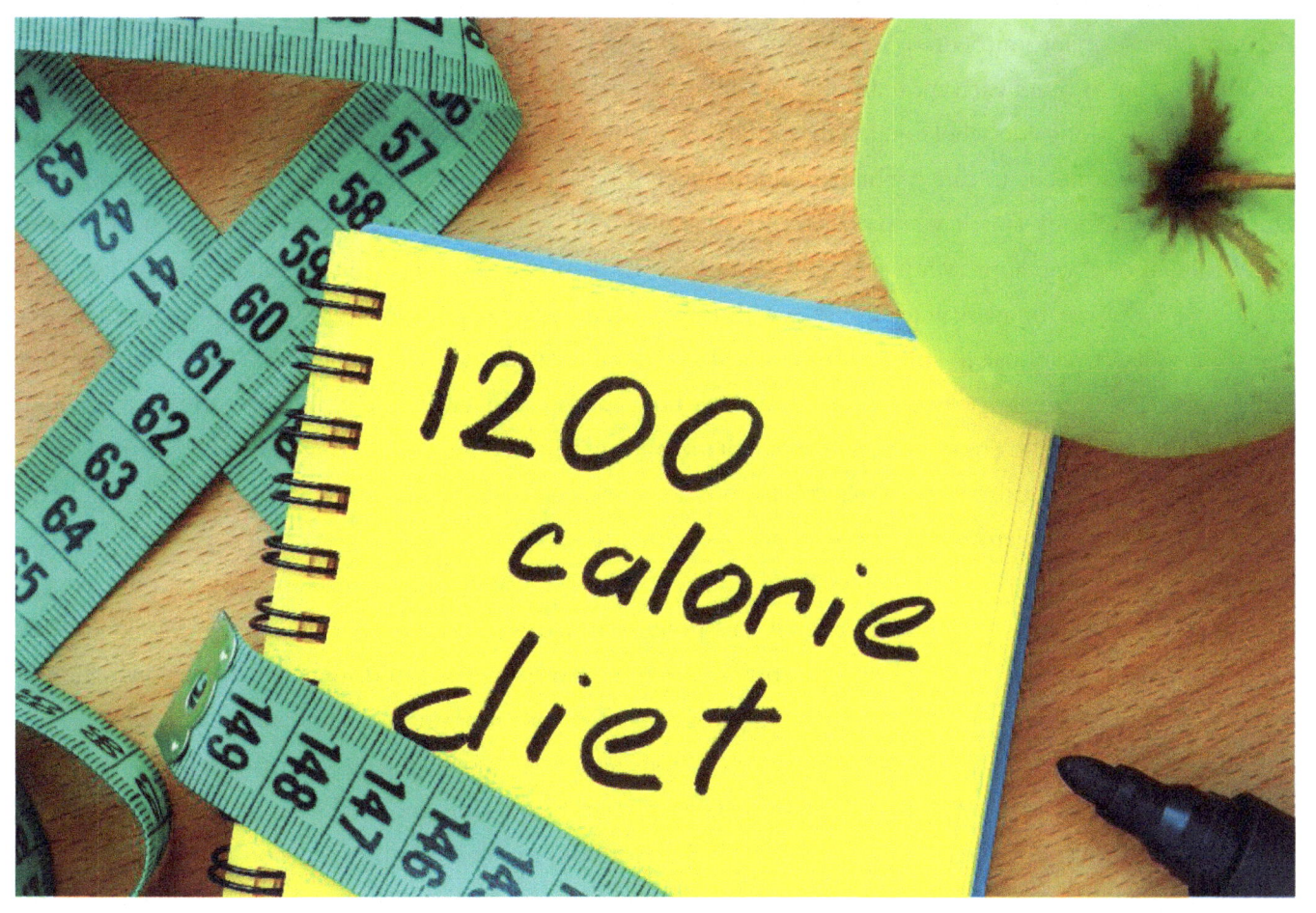

The core of Dr. Now's philosophy is built on three fundamental principles: calorie control, nutritional balance, and behavioral change. These principles work in harmony to create a comprehensive approach to weight loss that is not only effective but also sustainable in the long run.

Calorie control is the cornerstone of the Dr. Now approach. In a world where portion sizes have ballooned and convenience foods abound, it's easy to consume more calories than our bodies need. Dr. Now's plan addresses this by emphasizing the importance of maintaining a daily caloric intake that aligns with your weight loss goals. The plan typically centers around a 1200-calorie per day guideline, a number carefully chosen to ensure that you are consuming enough to meet your nutritional needs while still allowing for weight loss.

This concept may seem daunting at first, especially if you're used to eating more. However, it is not about deprivation but about making smarter choices. The idea is to maximize the nutritional value of every calorie you consume. By prioritizing whole, nutrient-dense foods, you can enjoy satisfying meals that leave you feeling full and energized. It's about eating more of the right things, rather than simply eating less.

The second pillar of the Dr. Now approach is nutritional balance. It's not enough to merely count calories; what matters is where those calories come from. The plan encourages a diet rich in lean proteins, complex carbohydrates, and healthy fats. These components provide the essential nutrients your body needs to function optimally and support weight loss. Lean proteins are a key component, as they help preserve muscle mass while you lose fat. Sources like chicken, fish, and plant-based proteins are not only filling but also versatile, allowing for a variety of delicious and satisfying meals. Complex carbohydrates, found in whole grains, fruits, and vegetables, provide sustained energy and help regulate blood sugar levels. Meanwhile, healthy fats from sources like nuts, seeds, and avocados are vital for brain health and hormone production.

Balancing these macronutrients is crucial for maintaining your health during weight loss. Dr. Now's plan encourages you to build each meal around a protein source and complement it with a colorful array of fruits and vegetables, alongside whole grains or starchy vegetables. This balance ensures that you are fueling your body with what it needs to thrive while keeping hunger at bay. The third and perhaps most critical element of Dr. Now's philosophy is behavioral change. Recognizing that weight loss is not just a physical challenge but also a mental one, the approach incorporates strategies to help you shift your mindset and develop healthier habits. It's about creating a new relationship with food, where eating becomes a mindful, intentional act rather than an impulsive response to stress or boredom. Behavioral change starts with awareness. By identifying your eating patterns and triggers, you can begin to address the root causes of overeating. Are you eating out of habit, or are you responding to emotional cues? Understanding the 'why' behind your eating habits is the first step in altering them. Dr. Now also emphasizes the importance of setting realistic, achievable goals. Success is built on a foundation of small victories that accumulate over time. It's about celebrating each step forward, no matter how minor it may seem. This approach helps to build confidence and momentum, keeping you motivated and committed to your goals. An integral part of this process is learning to practice mindfulness in eating. This involves paying attention to hunger cues, savoring each bite, and being present during meals. By slowing down and engaging fully with the experience of eating, you can enjoy your food more and prevent overeating.

Mindfulness also encourages you to listen to your body's signals, allowing you to stop eating when you're satisfied rather than stuffed. Another aspect of behavioral change is finding ways to incorporate physical activity into your daily routine. Exercise should not feel like a chore but rather a joyful expression of what your body can do. Whether it's a brisk walk, a dance class, or a yoga session, the key is to find activities that you enjoy and that fit into your lifestyle. Exercise not only aids in weight loss but also boosts mood, improves sleep, and enhances overall health. Support and accountability are also crucial components of the behavioral change process. Sharing your journey with friends, family, or a support group can provide encouragement and motivation. It's about having a network of people who understand your struggles and cheer your successes. This sense of community can make all the difference when you encounter challenges along the way.

Ultimately, the core philosophy of the Dr. Now approach is about empowerment. It's about equipping you with the knowledge and tools you need to take control of your health and your future. By focusing on calorie control, nutritional balance, and behavioral change, you can create a sustainable lifestyle that not only supports weight loss but also enhances your overall quality of life.

2. THE SCIENCE BEHIND THE DIET

Understanding the science behind the Dr. Now approach to dieting can illuminate why it is so effective and why it has worked for so many individuals seeking sustainable weight loss. At its core, the diet is designed around well-researched principles that focus on calorie reduction, macronutrient balance, and behavioral changes that align with how our bodies naturally function. The foundation of the Dr. Now diet lies in its approach to calorie restriction. To grasp this, we need to explore the basic principle of energy balance: the relationship between calories consumed and calories burned. Our bodies require a certain amount of energy to perform basic functions like breathing, circulating blood, and maintaining body temperature. This is known as our basal metabolic rate (BMR). Additionally, we need energy to fuel our daily activities, from walking and talking to more intense physical exercise.

Weight gain occurs when we consume more calories than we expend. This excess energy is stored in our bodies as fat. To lose weight, we need to create a calorie deficit, which means consuming fewer calories than our body needs. Dr. Now's 1200-calorie diet is structured to help achieve this deficit while still providing sufficient nutrients for health and vitality. Why 1200 calories, you might ask? For most people, this number is low enough to induce weight loss but high enough to prevent the body from going into starvation mode. When the body thinks it's starving, it can slow down metabolism and conserve energy, making it harder to lose weight. By carefully calibrating calorie intake, Dr. Now's approach ensures that weight loss is achievable and sustainable.

Another critical element of the Dr. Now diet is the focus on macronutrient balance. Our bodies require a combination of proteins, carbohydrates, and fats to function optimally. Proteins are essential for repairing and building tissues, making them crucial during weight loss to preserve muscle mass. Muscles burn more calories than fat, even at rest, so maintaining muscle mass is important for a healthy metabolism. Carbohydrates are our body's primary source of energy. However, not all carbs are created equal. The diet emphasizes complex carbohydrates, which are found in whole grains, fruits, and vegetables. These carbs are digested slowly, providing a steady release of energy and keeping blood sugar levels stable. Simple carbohydrates, found in sugary snacks and processed foods, are digested quickly, leading to energy spikes and crashes. Fats are often misunderstood in dieting, but they play a vital role in our health. They are necessary for the absorption of fat-soluble vitamins like A, D, E, and K, and they provide essential fatty acids that our bodies cannot produce on their own. The key is choosing healthy fats, such as those from avocados, nuts, and olive oil, while minimizing saturated and trans fats found in fried and processed foods.

A scientific understanding of insulin and blood sugar levels also underpins the Dr. Now approach. When we consume carbohydrates, our body breaks them down into glucose, which enters the bloodstream. The pancreas releases insulin, a hormone that helps cells absorb glucose for energy. However, consistently consuming high-glycemic foods can lead to insulin resistance, a condition where cells become less responsive to insulin. This resistance is a precursor to type 2 diabetes and can make weight loss more difficult.

By prioritizing low-glycemic foods that cause a slower rise in blood sugar, Dr. Now's diet helps maintain insulin sensitivity. This not only aids in weight loss but also supports overall health by reducing the risk of metabolic disorders. It's a scientific principle that brings clarity to why certain food choices are favored in the plan. Another crucial scientific aspect of the Dr. Now approach is understanding how our bodies use energy at rest versus during activity. Exercise is a powerful tool for weight loss, not only because it burns calories but also because it boosts metabolic rate. Engaging in regular physical activity increases muscle mass, which in turn enhances metabolism. The more lean muscle you have, the more calories you burn, even when you're not moving. However, exercise is only part of the equation. The plan recognizes that dietary changes have a more significant impact on weight loss than exercise alone. While movement is encouraged, the primary focus is on adopting a sustainable eating pattern that supports long-term weight management. Moreover, the Dr. Now approach incorporates an understanding of satiety and hunger hormones, such as leptin and ghrelin. Leptin is a hormone that signals satiety to the brain, helping us know when we're full. On the other hand, ghrelin, often referred to as the "hunger hormone," signals the brain when it's time to eat.

Dietary choices can influence these hormones. Consuming fiber-rich foods, for example, promotes satiety by slowing digestion and helping to regulate blood sugar levels. Protein is also known to increase the production of hormones that promote feelings of fullness, making it a cornerstone of the diet.

Lastly, the behavioral science behind the Dr. Now diet acknowledges the psychological aspects of eating and weight loss. Emotional and stress-related eating are common barriers to successful weight management. The plan encourages mindfulness and self-awareness, helping individuals recognize emotional triggers and develop healthier coping mechanisms. This psychological support is as important as the dietary guidelines, providing a holistic approach to weight loss.

3. Setting Realistic Goals

When starting out, the first step is to reflect on your motivations. Understanding why you want to lose weight can help you set goals that are meaningful and sustainable. Perhaps you want to improve your health markers, such as blood pressure or cholesterol levels, or maybe you aspire to have more energy to keep up with your children or grandchildren. Some people are motivated by the desire to feel more confident and comfortable in their own skin. Whatever your reason, knowing your "why" provides the foundation upon which your goals are built. Once you've identified your motivations, it's time to establish specific, measurable goals.

While it's tempting to focus solely on the number on the scale, it's important to remember that weight loss is not just about losing pounds. Instead, consider setting goals that encompass various aspects of your health and well-being. For instance, you might aim to increase your daily step count, improve your dietary habits, or develop a consistent exercise routine. These non-scale victories can provide a sense of achievement and boost your confidence as you progress.

One of the key principles of setting realistic goals is to break them down into smaller, manageable steps. Instead of aiming to lose a significant amount of weight in a short period, focus on achievable weekly or monthly targets. This approach not only makes your goals feel more attainable but also helps maintain motivation and momentum. Remember, progress is often incremental, and celebrating small wins along the way is vital for staying on track. Moreover, consider incorporating both short-term and long-term goals into your plan. Short-term goals provide immediate gratification and help you stay focused, while long-term goals offer a sense of direction and purpose. For example, a short-term goal might be to cook a healthy dinner three times a week, while a long-term goal could be to complete a 5K run or fit into a favorite outfit. By balancing these goals, you create a roadmap that guides you through your journey while allowing for flexibility and adaptation as needed. An essential aspect of setting realistic goals is to be kind to yourself. It's important to recognize that setbacks are a natural part of the process. There will be days when you miss a workout or indulge in a treat, and that's okay. Rather than viewing these moments as failures, see them as opportunities to learn and grow. Adjust your goals if necessary, and remember that perfection is not the aim. Progress, not perfection, is the true measure of success. Accountability can be a powerful motivator when working toward your goals. Share your objectives with a trusted friend, family member, or support group who can encourage you and hold you accountable. Having someone to share your triumphs and challenges with can provide the support and camaraderie needed to stay committed. Additionally, consider tracking your progress using a journal or an app. Recording your achievements and reflecting on your journey can boost your confidence and remind you of how far you've come. In setting your goals, it's also crucial to consider the broader lifestyle changes that accompany weight loss. The Dr. Now approach is not just about dieting; it's about transforming your relationship with food, exercise, and self-care. As you define your objectives, think about how you can integrate these changes into your daily life. This might involve meal planning, developing a morning routine, or finding activities you enjoy that keep you active. By aligning your goals with your lifestyle, you create a sustainable plan that supports lasting change. As you progress on your weight loss journey, be open to reassessing and adjusting your goals. Life is unpredictable, and circumstances can change. Flexibility is key to maintaining motivation and preventing frustration. If a goal no longer feels relevant or achievable, don't be afraid to pivot and set a new one. The journey to better health is not a straight line but rather a series of adjustments and recalibrations that reflect your evolving needs and priorities. Furthermore, consider the emotional and psychological aspects of weight loss. Setting goals that address these dimensions can enhance your overall well-being. For instance, you might set a goal to practice self-compassion or to spend time each week engaging in activities that bring you joy and relaxation. Weight loss is as much about nurturing the mind and spirit as it is about transforming the body. Incorporating mindfulness into your goal-setting process can also be beneficial. Take time to pause, reflect, and connect with your inner self. Mindfulness can help you tune into your body's signals, making you more aware of hunger cues and emotional triggers. By cultivating a sense of presence and awareness, you can make more intentional choices that align with your goals and values.

Ultimately, setting realistic goals is about creating a vision for your future self that is both inspiring and attainable. It's about believing in your ability to change and grow, even in the face of challenges. The Dr. Now approach empowers you to take control of your health and embrace the journey with confidence and resilience.

4. Customizing the Plan to Individual Needs

Adopting the Dr. Now approach to weight loss is like crafting a tailored suit—it's all about finding the perfect fit for you. Every individual is unique, with different lifestyles, preferences, and nutritional needs. Customizing the plan to suit your specific situation is key to ensuring not only effectiveness but also sustainability.

Think of this approach as a framework, a flexible guideline that can be adapted to fit your unique circumstances. The core principles remain the same: a focus on low-calorie, nutrient-dense foods, mindful eating, and balanced nutrition. However, the specifics of the plan can be adjusted to accommodate various factors such as dietary preferences, cultural influences, and health conditions. To begin customizing the plan, start by understanding your own dietary needs and goals. Are you aiming for weight loss, improved energy levels, or better overall health? Knowing your primary objective helps shape your approach and keeps you focused on what truly matters to you. It's also crucial to consider any dietary restrictions or allergies, ensuring that the foods you choose align with your health needs. Consider your lifestyle and daily schedule as you adapt the plan. Are you someone with a hectic work life, often finding yourself short on time for meal preparation? Or do you have the flexibility to experiment with new recipes and ingredients? Tailoring the plan to fit your lifestyle increases the likelihood of sticking with it. For those with limited time, focusing on quick, easy-to-prepare meals or embracing batch cooking can make a world of difference.

Cultural and personal food preferences also play a significant role in customizing the plan. Food is a deeply personal experience, often tied to cultural identity and family traditions. It's important to incorporate foods that you enjoy and that hold personal significance. This not only makes the plan more enjoyable but also more meaningful, enhancing your connection to the meals you prepare and consume.

Another aspect to consider is your level of physical activity. Are you someone who exercises regularly, or are you just starting to incorporate more movement into your routine? Your activity level can influence your nutritional needs, particularly in terms of protein intake and overall caloric requirements. Those engaging in more intense physical activity may require additional calories to support their energy expenditure and muscle recovery. Listening to your body is one of the most effective ways to customize your plan. Pay attention to how different foods make you feel, both physically and mentally. Do certain meals leave you feeling energized and satisfied, while others result in sluggishness or cravings? This self-awareness is invaluable, helping you identify which foods work best for you and which might need to be adjusted or replaced.

The emotional and psychological aspects of eating cannot be overlooked. Food is often tied to emotions, whether it's a source of comfort during stressful times or a way to celebrate special occasions. Understanding your emotional relationship with food can guide you in making more mindful choices. Perhaps stress leads to emotional eating, or social situations result in overindulgence. By recognizing these patterns, you can develop strategies to manage them more effectively. Accountability and support are critical components of a customized plan. Whether it's a friend, family member, or a professional like a dietitian, having someone to share your journey with can provide encouragement and motivation. They can offer insights, celebrate your successes, and provide guidance during challenging times.

This support system can be instrumental in maintaining long-term commitment and success. Experimentation is another valuable tool in the customization process. Don't be afraid to try new foods, recipes, or meal timings. This experimentation can reveal new favorites and open up a world of culinary possibilities that keep your meals exciting and diverse. It also allows you to adapt the plan as your tastes and needs evolve over time. Setting realistic and flexible goals is essential. While the ultimate aim may be significant weight loss or improved health metrics, breaking these goals down into smaller, achievable milestones can help maintain motivation. Celebrate these smaller victories along the way, recognizing that each step forward is progress, even if it doesn't always seem significant at the moment.

Lastly, remember that customization is an ongoing process. As you progress, your needs and circumstances may change. Stay attuned to these shifts and be willing to adapt your plan accordingly. Flexibility is key to ensuring that the plan remains effective and relevant, supporting you in reaching your goals while maintaining balance and enjoyment. Customizing the Dr. Now approach is about finding what works best for you as an individual. It's about honoring your preferences, respecting your limitations, and embracing your potential. By crafting a plan that aligns with your unique needs, you set the stage for a successful and sustainable journey toward better health and well-being. Trust in your ability to make informed choices and create a plan that not only supports your goals but also enhances your quality of life.

5. Psychological Aspects of Dieting

Dieting is as much a mental journey as it is a physical one. Understanding the psychological aspects of dieting can be the key to unlocking lasting success and fostering a healthier relationship with food. As we delve into the intricacies of the mind and its influence on our eating habits, we begin to see the profound impact that thoughts, emotions, and beliefs have on our dietary choices and outcomes. At the heart of successful dieting is the ability to cultivate a positive mindset. This begins with self-awareness, a critical tool in recognizing our thought patterns and emotional triggers related to food. Often, we eat not just out of hunger but in response to emotions such as stress, boredom, or sadness. These emotional eating patterns can sabotage our best intentions, leading to overeating and weight gain. By becoming aware of these triggers, we can begin to develop strategies to address them, such as finding alternative coping mechanisms or practicing mindfulness. Mindfulness, in particular, is a powerful tool in the realm of dieting. It involves paying full attention to the present moment, allowing us to become more attuned to our body's hunger and satiety signals. When we eat mindfully, we savor each bite, appreciating the flavors and textures of our food. This practice not only enhances our enjoyment of meals but also helps prevent overeating by encouraging us to stop when we are comfortably full rather than mindlessly consuming food. The beliefs we hold about food and our bodies also play a significant role in the psychological landscape of dieting. Many of us carry deep-seated beliefs about what foods are "good" or "bad," often shaped by societal norms and past experiences. These beliefs can lead to guilt or shame when we eat certain foods, which in turn can trigger emotional eating or restrictive dieting practices. Challenging these beliefs and adopting a more balanced perspective can be liberating, allowing us to enjoy a variety of foods without judgment or fear. Self-talk is another crucial aspect of the psychological journey. The way we speak to ourselves about our bodies and our dietary choices can either empower or undermine our efforts. Negative self-talk, such as "I'll never be able to stick to this diet" or "I'm so bad for eating that dessert," can erode our confidence and motivation. On the other hand, positive affirmations and compassionate self-talk can bolster our resolve and foster resilience. Reminding ourselves of our strengths, acknowledging our efforts, and celebrating small victories can create a supportive internal dialogue that encourages perseverance. The role of motivation in dieting cannot be overstated. Understanding why we want to make changes to our diet is crucial in maintaining long-term commitment. Motivation can stem from a variety of sources, such as the desire for improved health, increased energy, or enhanced self-esteem. By identifying our core motivations, we can keep these reasons at the forefront of our minds, especially during challenging times. Visualizing the outcomes we desire and how they will positively impact our lives can serve as a powerful motivator, propelling us forward even when the journey feels arduous.

Social influences also play a significant role in the psychological aspects of dieting. Our social circles, including family, friends, and coworkers, can either support or hinder our dietary efforts. While some may offer encouragement and share in our journey, others might unknowingly undermine our goals through peer pressure or skepticism. Navigating these dynamics requires clear communication and, at times, setting boundaries to protect our progress. Surrounding ourselves with a supportive network, whether in person or through online communities, can provide a sense of camaraderie and shared purpose.

Goal-setting is a practical strategy that bridges the psychological and practical aspects of dieting. Setting specific, achievable goals provides direction and a sense of purpose. It allows us to measure our progress and celebrate milestones along the way. However, it's important to set realistic expectations and to be flexible in our approach. Life is unpredictable, and being adaptable in the face of setbacks or challenges is key to maintaining motivation and commitment. Stress management is another critical component of the psychological approach to dieting. Stress can significantly impact our eating habits, often leading to emotional eating or poor food choices. Developing effective stress management techniques, such as exercise, meditation, or creative pursuits, can help mitigate these effects. By reducing stress, we create an environment that supports healthier eating habits and overall well-being. Finally, the psychological journey of dieting involves embracing self-compassion. It's easy to be critical of ourselves when we stumble or deviate from our plan, but it's important to remember that setbacks are a natural part of the process. By treating ourselves with kindness and understanding, we can maintain a positive outlook and the resilience needed to continue our journey. Embracing imperfection and viewing challenges as opportunities for growth can transform our relationship with food and ourselves. In conclusion, the psychological aspects of dieting are integral to achieving lasting success. By cultivating a positive mindset, challenging limiting beliefs, and developing strategies to manage stress and emotions, we can create a supportive environment for change. The journey is as much about transforming our relationship with food and our bodies as it is about the numbers on the scale. With mindfulness, self-awareness, and compassion, we can navigate the complexities of dieting and emerge stronger, healthier, and more empowered.

CHAPTER 2: THE POWER OF NUTRITION
1. HEALTH BENEFITS OF EATING RIGHT

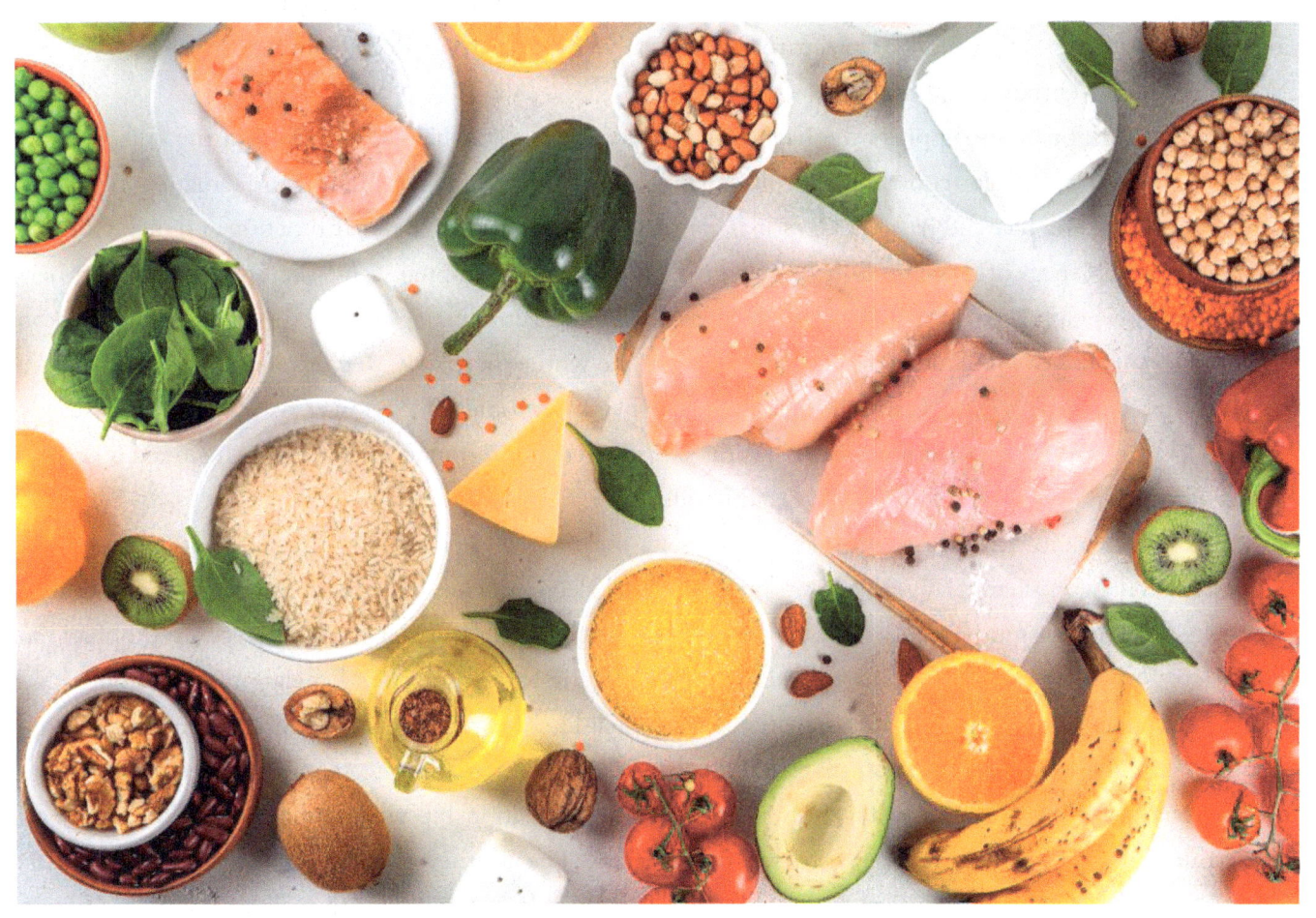

At the heart of healthy eating is the prevention of chronic diseases. Conditions such as heart disease, diabetes, and certain cancers are often linked to dietary choices. By prioritizing a diet rich in fruits, vegetables, whole grains, and lean proteins, you provide your body with the nutrients it needs to function optimally. These foods are packed with vitamins, minerals, antioxidants, and fiber, all of which play a crucial role in maintaining health and preventing disease. For instance, a diet high in fiber helps regulate blood sugar levels, reduces cholesterol, and supports digestive health. Fiber is found abundantly in foods like oats, beans, and fruits, and it has the added benefit of promoting satiety, helping you feel full and satisfied after meals. This can be particularly beneficial for those working toward weight loss goals, as it helps control hunger and reduce the likelihood of overeating. Antioxidants, found in colorful fruits and vegetables such as berries, leafy greens, and bell peppers, are another vital component of a healthy diet. They protect your cells from damage caused by free radicals, unstable molecules that can contribute to the development of chronic diseases. By neutralizing these free radicals, antioxidants help reduce inflammation, support the immune system, and slow the aging process. In addition to preventing disease, eating right can significantly improve your mental health. There is a growing body of research highlighting the connection between nutrition and mental well-being. Certain nutrients, like omega-3 fatty acids found in fish, are known to support brain health and can reduce symptoms of depression and anxiety. Similarly, complex carbohydrates found in whole grains promote the production of serotonin, a neurotransmitter that enhances mood and promotes feelings of well-being. The benefits of healthy eating extend to energy levels and cognitive function. Consuming a balanced diet provides a steady supply of energy throughout the day, helping you stay alert and focused. The brain relies on glucose for fuel, and eating complex carbohydrates ensures a gradual release of glucose into the bloodstream, avoiding the spikes and crashes associated with sugary snacks and refined carbs. This steady energy supply not only improves productivity but also enhances concentration and memory.

Moreover, a nutritious diet supports the health of your skin, hair, and nails. Vitamins and minerals such as vitamin C, vitamin E, and zinc contribute to collagen production and skin repair, leading to a radiant complexion and stronger, healthier hair and nails. Hydration is also crucial, as it supports cellular function and maintains the elasticity and suppleness of the skin. Drinking plenty of water and consuming water-rich foods like cucumbers and watermelon helps keep your skin hydrated and glowing. Healthy eating also has a profound impact on longevity and quality of life. Studies have shown that people who adhere to a Mediterranean-style diet, rich in fruits, vegetables, whole grains, and healthy fats, tend to live longer and have a lower risk of chronic diseases. This way of eating promotes cardiovascular health, supports cognitive function, and helps maintain a healthy weight, all of which contribute to a longer, healthier life.

One of the lesser-known benefits of eating right is its impact on sleep quality. Certain nutrients, such as magnesium and tryptophan, play a role in promoting restful sleep. Magnesium, found in nuts, seeds, and leafy greens, helps relax the muscles and calm the nervous system, making it easier to fall asleep. Tryptophan, an amino acid found in turkey and dairy products, is a precursor to serotonin and melatonin, hormones that regulate sleep cycles. As you embrace a nutritious diet, you'll likely notice a positive shift in your relationship with food. Rather than viewing it as an adversary or a source of guilt, you begin to see food as nourishment and fuel for your body. This mindset change can lead to a healthier relationship with eating, where you savor and enjoy your meals rather than feeling restricted or deprived. The journey to eating right is not without its challenges, but the rewards far outweigh the obstacles. It requires a commitment to making informed choices and a willingness to experiment with new foods and recipes. It also involves a degree of planning and preparation to ensure that healthy options are readily available, especially during busy or stressful times. Building a healthy eating routine often starts with small, manageable changes. This might mean adding an extra serving of vegetables to your dinner or swapping a sugary snack for a piece of fruit. Over time, these small adjustments can lead to significant improvements in your health and well-being. The key is to focus on progress, not perfection, and to celebrate the positive changes you're making along the way. Incorporating mindfulness into your eating habits can further enhance the benefits of a nutritious diet. Mindful eating involves paying attention to your hunger cues, savoring each bite, and being fully present during meals. This practice not only helps prevent overeating but also encourages you to appreciate the flavors and textures of your food, leading to greater satisfaction and enjoyment.

2. COMMON NUTRITIONAL PITFALLS

One of the most prevalent nutritional pitfalls is the allure of "quick-fix" diets. In our fast-paced world, the promise of rapid weight loss can be incredibly tempting. Diets that promise dramatic results in a short time often gain popularity quickly, fueled by testimonials and sensational headlines. However, these diets often involve extreme calorie restriction or the elimination of entire food groups, which can be detrimental to your health. While you may see quick results initially, these diets are rarely sustainable, and the weight often returns once normal eating patterns resume. Another common mistake is falling for marketing labels that give the illusion of health. Terms like "natural," "low-fat," "sugar-free," and "organic" can be misleading, making it difficult to discern what is genuinely beneficial. For example, many "low-fat" products compensate for reduced fat by adding sugar, which can contribute to weight gain and other health issues. It's essential to read nutrition labels carefully, paying attention to ingredients and nutritional content rather than relying solely on marketing claims. Portion distortion is another pitfall that many people encounter. Over the years, portion sizes have increased dramatically, both in restaurants and at home. What we perceive as a normal serving size today is often much larger than it should be. This distortion leads to unintentional overeating, even when we think we're making healthy choices. Learning to recognize appropriate portion sizes and being mindful of how much we're eating can help mitigate this issue. Another challenge is the reliance on convenience foods, which often contain high levels of sodium, sugar, and unhealthy fats. While convenience foods can be a lifesaver on busy days, they should not form the cornerstone of your diet. Preparing meals at home using whole, unprocessed ingredients allows you to control what goes into your food and helps ensure you're getting the nutrients you need. When time is short, consider preparing meals in advance or opting for healthier convenience options like pre-washed salads or rotisserie chicken. Emotional eating is a pitfall that many people struggle with. Food is often used as a coping mechanism for dealing with stress, sadness, or boredom. While it may provide temporary comfort, emotional eating can lead to unhealthy habits and weight gain over time. Developing strategies to manage emotions without turning to food, such as engaging in physical activity, practicing mindfulness, or seeking support from friends and family, can help break this cycle.

The misconception that all calories are created equal is another common pitfall. While it's true that calories are a measure of energy, the source of those calories matters significantly. A calorie from a sugary drink is not equivalent to a calorie from a piece of fruit. Foods rich in nutrients provide the vitamins, minerals, and fiber your body needs to function optimally, while empty calories offer little more than energy, often leading to cravings and overeating. Prioritizing nutrient-dense foods ensures that your body receives the fuel it needs without unnecessary additives.

Skipping meals, especially breakfast, is a habit that many fall into, often in the name of saving calories. However, skipping meals can backfire, leading to increased hunger and overeating later in the day. Eating regular, balanced meals helps maintain steady energy levels and prevents the temptation to reach for unhealthy snacks. Breakfast, in particular, is an opportunity to kickstart your metabolism and provide your body with the energy it needs to start the day. Fad diets that promote extreme restrictions or demonize certain food groups are another common trap. Carbohydrates, for example, have been unfairly vilified in some diet trends. While it's important to be mindful of carbohydrate choices, completely eliminating them can deprive your body of essential nutrients and energy. Similarly, diets that eliminate fats can miss out on the benefits of healthy fats, which are crucial for brain health and hormone production. A balanced diet that includes a variety of foods in moderation is the key to long-term success. Another pitfall is not drinking enough water. Hydration is often overlooked in the pursuit of health, yet it is vital for every bodily function. Water helps regulate temperature, transport nutrients, and remove waste. Dehydration can lead to fatigue, headaches, and impaired concentration, often mistaken for hunger, leading to unnecessary snacking. Keeping a water bottle handy and making a conscious effort to drink regularly throughout the day can support overall health and prevent mistaking thirst for hunger. Not all supplements are created equal, and relying too heavily on them can be a nutritional pitfall.

While supplements can be beneficial in certain situations, they should not replace whole foods. The nutrients found in whole foods are often more bioavailable and work synergistically with other compounds in the food to provide maximum benefit. It's best to focus on obtaining nutrients from a varied and balanced diet, using supplements only to fill specific gaps as recommended by a healthcare professional.

Finally, neglecting to listen to your body's signals is a common mistake. In the quest to follow diets or meet specific calorie goals, it's easy to overlook hunger and fullness cues. Each person's body is unique, and learning to listen to your own hunger and satiety signals is crucial for developing a healthy relationship with food. Mindful eating practices can help you become more attuned to these signals, allowing you to eat when you're hungry and stop when you're satisfied.

3. BUILDING A BALANCED DIET

To begin building a balanced diet, it's essential to understand the role of macronutrients: proteins, carbohydrates, and fats. Each macronutrient serves a specific purpose and contributes to your overall health. Proteins are the building blocks of your body, responsible for repairing tissues, producing enzymes, and supporting immune function. They provide the necessary amino acids that help build muscle, strengthen hair and nails, and promote healthy skin. Carbohydrates, often misunderstood in modern diets, are your body's primary energy source. They fuel your brain, muscles, and other organs, enabling you to perform both physical and mental tasks. Carbohydrates should primarily come from complex sources like whole grains, fruits, and vegetables, which offer sustained energy release and are packed with fiber, vitamins, and minerals. Fats, once feared as a dietary villain, are vital for absorbing fat-soluble vitamins (A, D, E, and K), protecting organs, and maintaining cell membranes. Healthy fats, found in avocados, nuts, seeds, and olive oil, support brain health, hormone production, and inflammation reduction. Striking the right balance among these macronutrients is key to supporting energy levels, metabolic function, and overall well-being.

A balanced diet should also include a variety of micronutrients, such as vitamins and minerals, which play numerous roles in maintaining health. These nutrients are involved in bone health, nerve function, immune support, and countless other bodily processes. Consuming a wide range of colorful fruits and vegetables ensures that you receive an array of essential vitamins and minerals. For instance, dark leafy greens like spinach and kale are rich in iron and calcium, while citrus fruits provide ample vitamin C.

When constructing a balanced diet, consider the importance of portion control and moderation. Even nutritious foods can contribute to weight gain if consumed in excess. Learning to listen to your body's hunger and fullness cues is essential. Practicing mindful eating—savoring each bite, eating slowly, and paying attention to satiety signals—can help you develop a healthier relationship with food.

One practical way to visualize a balanced diet is through the plate method. Imagine your plate divided into sections: half filled with colorful vegetables and fruits, a quarter with lean protein, and a quarter with whole grains. This method ensures a variety of nutrients and promotes portion control, making it easier to create balanced meals without the need for complicated calculations or rigid rules. Variety is another cornerstone of a balanced diet. Eating a wide range of foods ensures that you receive all the nutrients your body needs. Different foods provide different nutrients, and no single food can supply everything your body requires. Experiment with new foods and flavors, exploring different cuisines and cooking methods to keep your meals interesting and enjoyable. Embracing variety can also help prevent dietary monotony, which often leads to cravings for less healthy options. Hydration is an often-overlooked aspect of a balanced diet but is essential for health. Water is involved in nearly every bodily function, from regulating temperature and transporting nutrients to flushing out waste products. Aim to drink enough water throughout the day to keep your body hydrated and functioning optimally. Herbal teas and water-rich fruits and vegetables, like cucumbers and melons, can also contribute to your daily fluid intake. Building a balanced diet is not only about what you eat but also about how you eat. The social and emotional aspects of eating are important components of a healthy diet. Sharing meals with family and friends, enjoying food without distraction, and taking time to prepare and appreciate your food can enhance the eating experience and support your overall well-being.

Incorporating physical activity into your routine complements a balanced diet and contributes to a healthy lifestyle. Exercise supports weight management, boosts mood, improves cardiovascular health, and strengthens muscles and bones. Aim for a mix of aerobic activities, strength training, and flexibility exercises to achieve a well-rounded fitness regimen that supports your dietary efforts. Remember, building a balanced diet is not about strict restrictions or depriving yourself of the foods you love. It's about creating a sustainable pattern of eating that supports your health goals and enhances your quality of life. This approach allows for occasional indulgences while maintaining overall balance. By focusing on nutrient-dense foods and listening to your body's needs, you can enjoy a wide variety of flavors and textures while nourishing your body.

4. Essential Nutrients and Where to Find Them

In the vibrant world of nutrition, essential nutrients stand as the building blocks of health and vitality. These nutrients are indispensable, playing crucial roles in maintaining bodily functions and supporting overall well-being. Understanding what these nutrients are and where to find them empowers us to make informed choices that nourish our bodies and enhance our quality of life.

The body relies on six primary categories of essential nutrients: carbohydrates, proteins, fats, vitamins, minerals, and water. Each of these nutrients fulfills specific functions and contributes to the intricate tapestry of life. They work in harmony, supporting growth, energy production, immune function, and countless other processes that keep us healthy and thriving. Carbohydrates are the body's main source of energy, fueling everything from breathing to exercising. They are broken down into glucose, which powers our cells, tissues, and organs. Carbohydrates can be found in a variety of foods, including fruits, vegetables, grains, and legumes. These foods not only provide energy but also deliver dietary fiber, which aids digestion and helps maintain stable blood sugar levels. Proteins are the building blocks of the body, involved in the creation of tissues, enzymes, hormones, and antibodies. They play a vital role in repairing and maintaining body structures. Protein can be sourced from both animal and plant foods, including meat, fish, eggs, dairy, beans, lentils, and nuts. Ensuring an adequate intake of protein is crucial for maintaining muscle mass and supporting immune function.

Fats, often misunderstood, are essential for absorbing fat-soluble vitamins, protecting organs, and providing long-term energy storage. They are categorized into saturated, unsaturated, and trans fats, each with different effects on health. Healthy fats, such as those found in avocados, olive oil, nuts, and seeds, contribute to heart health and reduce inflammation. Balancing fat intake is important for achieving optimal health and avoiding excesses that can lead to chronic diseases. Vitamins are organic compounds that are crucial for various metabolic processes. They support immune function, aid in the production of energy, and protect against oxidative stress. Each vitamin serves specific functions; for example, vitamin C boosts immunity, vitamin D supports bone health, and vitamin E acts as an antioxidant. Fruits, vegetables, and fortified foods are excellent sources of vitamins, offering a colorful and varied palette of options to meet our needs.

Minerals, like vitamins, are critical for a wide array of bodily functions. They help build strong bones and teeth, carry out nerve impulses, and regulate muscle function. Key minerals include calcium, potassium, iron, and magnesium. These can be found in foods such as dairy products, leafy greens, nuts, seeds, and whole grains. Ensuring a diverse and balanced diet helps provide the essential minerals necessary for maintaining health. Water, the elixir of life, is essential for every cell, tissue, and organ in the body. It facilitates digestion, aids in nutrient absorption, and regulates body temperature. While we often focus on what we eat, what we drink is equally important. Staying hydrated is vital for overall health, and water should be the primary beverage of choice. Consuming water-rich foods, like cucumbers and watermelon, can also contribute to hydration. The synergy between these nutrients is a testament to the complexity and brilliance of human biology. Each nutrient complements the others, working together to sustain life. For example, vitamin C enhances iron absorption, while calcium and vitamin D collaborate to promote bone health. Understanding these interactions can help guide dietary choices and optimize nutrient intake. Our nutritional needs can change throughout our lives, influenced by factors such as age, activity level, and health status. For example, athletes may require more protein to support muscle repair, while older adults may need increased calcium to maintain bone density. Recognizing these needs and adjusting our diets accordingly ensures that we continue to meet our nutritional requirements. In our quest to meet these needs, whole foods stand out as the best sources of essential nutrients. These foods are minimally processed, rich in vitamins, minerals, and other beneficial compounds. They provide a wealth of nutrition without the added sugars, unhealthy fats, and preservatives found in many processed foods. By focusing on whole foods, we can nourish our bodies naturally and effectively.

A varied diet is the key to obtaining a broad spectrum of nutrients. Different foods offer different nutrients, and incorporating a wide array of colors, flavors, and textures can help ensure comprehensive nutrition. Eating seasonally and locally not only enhances freshness and taste but also supports sustainable food systems. While supplements can help fill nutritional gaps, they should not replace a healthy diet. Whole foods offer more than isolated nutrients; they provide a complex matrix of compounds that work together to promote health. Supplements can be beneficial in certain situations, such as pregnancy or specific nutrient deficiencies, but they should be used wisely and under the guidance of a healthcare professional. Nutrition is an ever-evolving field, and staying informed about the latest research and recommendations is important. As we learn more about the impact of nutrition on health, we can make adjustments to our diets that reflect current understanding and best practices. This ongoing journey of discovery enriches our lives and empowers us to take charge of our health. Ultimately, the power of nutrition lies in its ability to transform our well-being. By understanding and embracing the essential nutrients and where to find them, we can make informed choices that support a vibrant, healthy life. It is a journey of exploration and empowerment, where each meal becomes an opportunity to nourish and energize our bodies. With knowledge and intention, we can harness the power of nutrition to enhance our health and enrich our lives.

5. ANTI-INFLAMMATORY FOODS FOR LONGEVITY

In the quest for longevity and optimal health, the role of inflammation in the body has come under intense scrutiny. While inflammation is a natural and essential process that helps the body heal and fight infections, chronic inflammation can contribute to a host of health issues, including heart disease, diabetes, cancer, and neurodegenerative disorders. Understanding how diet influences inflammation is crucial in promoting health and extending lifespan.

At the heart of this understanding is the recognition that certain foods have the power to reduce inflammation and enhance well-being. These anti-inflammatory foods are not just beneficial for immediate health but also hold the promise of longevity, helping to maintain vitality and prevent age-related diseases. Imagine your body as a finely tuned machine. Just as a car requires regular maintenance and quality fuel to run efficiently, your body thrives on nutrients that reduce inflammation and support optimal functioning. Anti-inflammatory foods act as high-quality fuel, providing the essential nutrients needed to keep your body's systems running smoothly and efficiently. Fruits and vegetables are the cornerstone of an anti-inflammatory diet. They are rich in vitamins, minerals, antioxidants, and phytochemicals, all of which play a crucial role in combating inflammation. Berries, for instance, are packed with antioxidants such as anthocyanins, which help reduce oxidative stress and inflammation. Leafy greens like spinach and kale are abundant in vitamins and minerals, supporting immune function and cellular health. The vibrant colors of these foods are a testament to their nutrient density and anti-inflammatory potential. Healthy fats, particularly those found in nuts, seeds, avocados, and fatty fish, are powerful allies in the fight against inflammation. Omega-3 fatty acids, prevalent in fish such as salmon, mackerel, and sardines, are renowned for their anti-inflammatory properties. They help balance the body's inflammatory response, supporting heart health and reducing the risk of chronic diseases. Incorporating these fats into your diet not only benefits inflammation but also provides essential nutrients that support brain function and mood. Whole grains, as opposed to refined grains, offer significant anti-inflammatory benefits. They are rich in fiber, which supports gut health and helps regulate the body's inflammatory processes. Foods like quinoa, brown rice, and oats are excellent choices, providing sustained energy and contributing to a balanced diet. The fiber in whole grains also aids in maintaining a healthy weight, which is crucial for reducing inflammation.

Herbs and spices are another potent source of anti-inflammatory compounds. Turmeric, with its active ingredient curcumin, is one of the most powerful natural anti-inflammatories. It has been extensively studied for its ability to combat chronic inflammation and is believed to play a role in preventing degenerative diseases. Ginger, garlic, and cinnamon also offer anti-inflammatory benefits, enhancing both flavor and health in your meals. Incorporating a variety of these foods into your diet can significantly impact your overall health and longevity. It's about creating a dietary pattern that consistently includes these nutrient-rich foods, supporting your body's natural ability to manage inflammation and repair itself. This approach is not about restriction but about abundance—focusing on the rich tapestry of flavors and nutrients that nature provides.

Hydration is an often-overlooked aspect of managing inflammation. Adequate water intake supports every bodily function, including those that regulate inflammation. Herbal teas, such as green tea and chamomile, offer additional anti-inflammatory compounds while contributing to hydration. Green tea, in particular, contains polyphenols that are known for their powerful anti-inflammatory and antioxidant effects. The balance of your diet is crucial. While adding anti-inflammatory foods is beneficial, it's equally important to minimize pro-inflammatory foods. Processed foods high in sugar, refined carbohydrates, and unhealthy fats can exacerbate inflammation and should be consumed sparingly. By focusing on whole, unprocessed foods, you can create a diet that supports your health and longevity. The impact of anti-inflammatory foods extends beyond physical health. Chronic inflammation is linked to mood disorders and cognitive decline, and reducing inflammation can improve mental clarity and emotional well-being. By nourishing your body with anti-inflammatory foods, you can support both physical and mental health, enhancing your quality of life. The journey towards incorporating more anti-inflammatory foods is an opportunity to explore new flavors and cooking methods. It invites creativity in the kitchen, encouraging experimentation with new ingredients and dishes. This exploration not only supports health but also brings joy and satisfaction to your meals, transforming eating into a celebration of nourishment and wellness.

As you embrace an anti-inflammatory diet, it's important to remember that lifestyle factors also play a role in managing inflammation. Regular physical activity, adequate sleep, and stress management techniques such as meditation and yoga complement dietary changes, creating a holistic approach to health. Together, these practices foster a balanced lifestyle that supports longevity and vitality. In conclusion, anti-inflammatory foods are a powerful tool in the pursuit of long-term health and longevity. They offer protection against chronic diseases, enhance physical and mental well-being, and provide the nutrients necessary for a vibrant life. By choosing to focus on these foods, you are taking proactive steps towards nurturing your body, supporting its natural functions, and paving the way for a healthier, more fulfilling future. Embrace the power of nutrition as a means to live not only longer but better, with vitality and vigor.

CHAPTER 3: THE 90-DAY MEAL PLAN
1. Introduction to the Meal Plan

Imagine this meal plan as your personal guide, offering a structured yet flexible framework to help you navigate the complexities of nutrition. It's crafted to suit diverse needs and preferences, recognizing that there is no one-size-fits-all solution when it comes to diet and health. The goal is to provide a foundation that empowers you to make informed choices, experiment with new foods, and develop a routine that fits seamlessly into your life. The beauty of this plan lies in its simplicity. It's built around whole, unprocessed foods that nourish your body and keep you feeling satisfied. By focusing on lean proteins, healthy fats, and complex carbohydrates, it provides the energy you need to tackle your day while keeping hunger at bay. The plan emphasizes balance, ensuring you receive the right mix of macronutrients and micronutrients to support your body's functions. Throughout these 90 days, you'll discover the power of variety. Eating a wide range of foods not only ensures you get all the nutrients your body needs but also keeps your meals exciting. Think of it as a culinary adventure, where each week brings new flavors and textures to explore. From hearty breakfasts to satisfying dinners, the plan is designed to prevent monotony and keep your taste buds engaged. A key component of the meal plan is meal prepping. Preparing your meals in advance can save you time and stress during busy weeks. It helps you stay on track by ensuring you always have healthy options on hand, reducing the temptation to reach for convenient but unhealthy alternatives. As you become more familiar with meal prepping, you'll find it becomes an integral part of your routine, simplifying your life and supporting your goals. While the plan provides a structured approach, it also allows for flexibility. Life is unpredictable, and there will be days when sticking to the plan feels challenging. The key is to be adaptable and give yourself grace. If a day doesn't go as planned, remember that it's just one day in a 90-day journey. The focus should be on progress, not perfection. Allow yourself the occasional indulgence without guilt, knowing that you can return to your healthy habits the next day. Hydration plays a vital role in this plan. Water is essential for every bodily function, from digestion to circulation. Ensuring you drink enough water each day helps you feel energized and can even aid in weight loss by preventing overeating. Herbal teas and infused waters are great options to keep things interesting if plain water feels monotonous. Another important aspect of the meal plan is mindfulness. Being present and aware while eating can enhance your enjoyment of food and prevent overeating. Take the time to savor each bite, appreciating the flavors and textures. This practice not only helps with portion control but also strengthens your connection with your body's hunger and fullness cues. Community support can be a valuable asset during these 90 days. Sharing your journey with friends, family, or online groups can provide encouragement and accountability. It's an opportunity to exchange tips, celebrate victories, and seek advice during challenging times. Having a support system can make the journey more enjoyable and help you stay committed to your goals. Tracking your progress is another useful tool. While the scale can provide some feedback, it's not the only measure of success. Consider tracking other indicators, such as energy levels, mood, sleep quality, and how your clothes fit. These non-scale victories can offer a more comprehensive view of your progress and keep you motivated. Remember, the ultimate goal of this meal plan is to cultivate a sustainable lifestyle that supports your health and well-being. It's about making gradual changes that become permanent habits, creating a foundation for long-term success. As you move through these 90 days, embrace the journey with curiosity and openness, knowing that each step you take is bringing you closer to a healthier, more vibrant life.

Scan the QR code below to download and print your very own meal plan.

Get started on your delicious journey!

CHAPTER 4: BREAKFAST OPTIONS

1. QUICK AND EASY RECIPES

SPINACH AND FETA BREAKFAST WRAP

P.T.: 5 min.
C.T.: 5 min.
M.C: Stovetop
SERVINGS: 1
INGR:
- 1 whole-grain tortilla
- 1 Cup fresh spinach
- 1/4 Cup crumbled feta cheese
- 2 large eggs
- 1 Tbsp olive oil
- Salt and pepper to taste

DIRECTIONS:
1. Heat olive oil in a skillet over medium heat.
2. Add spinach to the skillet and sauté until wilted.
3. In a bowl, whisk eggs with salt and pepper.
4. Pour eggs into the skillet with spinach and cook until set.
5. Sprinkle feta cheese over the eggs and cook until slightly melted.
6. Place the egg mixture onto the tortilla, wrap tightly, and serve immediately.

TIPS:
- Add a dash of hot sauce for extra flavor.
- Serve with a side of fresh fruit for a balanced meal.

N.V.: Calories: 320, Fat: 22g, Carbs: 20g, Protein: 18g, Sugar: 1g

AVOCADO TOAST WITH POACHED EGG

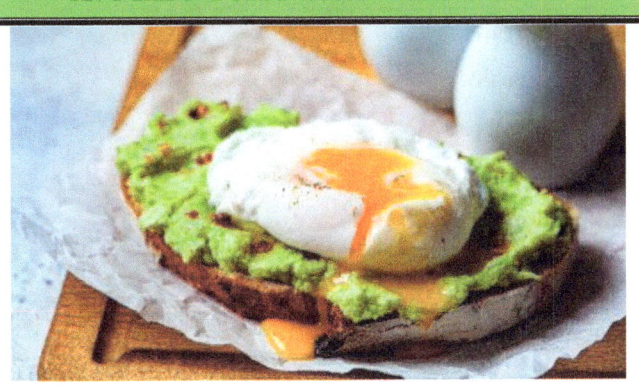

P.T.: 5 min.
C.T.: 5 min.
M.C: Stovetop
SERVINGS: 1
INGR:
- 1 slice whole-grain bread
- 1/2 ripe avocado
- 1 large egg
- 1 Tsp white vinegar
- Salt and pepper to taste
- Red pepper flakes (optional)

DIRECTIONS:
1. Toast the bread until golden brown.
2. Mash the avocado with salt and pepper, then spread it on the toast.
3. Bring a small pot of water to a gentle simmer and add vinegar.
4. Crack the egg into a bowl and gently slide it into the simmering water.
5. Cook for 3 minutes, then remove with a slotted spoon and place on avocado toast.
6. Sprinkle with red pepper flakes if desired and serve immediately.

TIPS:
- Use a fresh egg for the best poaching results.
- Garnish with microgreens for a nutritional boost.

N.V.: Calories: 250, Fat: 18g, Carbs: 20g, Protein: 10g, Sugar: 1g

BANANA OATMEAL PANCAKES

P.T.: 5 min.
C.T.: 10 min.
M.C: Stovetop
SERVINGS: 2
INGR:
- 1 Cup rolled oats
- 1 ripe banana
- 2 large eggs
- 1/4 Cup milk
- 1 Tsp baking powder
- 1/2 Tsp vanilla extract
- 1 Tbsp coconut oil

DIRECTIONS:
1. Blend oats in a food processor until fine.
2. Add banana, eggs, milk, baking powder, and vanilla extract to the oats and blend until smooth.
3. Heat coconut oil in a skillet over medium heat.
4. Pour batter onto the skillet, forming small pancakes.
5. Cook until bubbles form on the surface, then flip and cook until golden brown.
6. Serve with additional banana slices or a drizzle of maple syrup.

TIPS:
- Add a pinch of cinnamon for extra flavor.
- Use almond milk for a dairy-free option.

N.V.: Calories: 350, Fat: 12g, Carbs: 50g, Protein: 10g, Sugar: 12g

SMOKED SALMON AND CREAM CHEESE BAGEL

P.T.: 5 min.
C.T.: 0 min.
M.C: None
SERVINGS: 1
INGR:
- 1 whole-grain bagel
- 2 oz smoked salmon
- 2 Tbsp cream cheese
- 1 slice red onion
- 1 slice tomato
- Capers (optional)

DIRECTIONS:
1. Slice the bagel in half and toast until golden brown.
2. Spread cream cheese evenly on each half of the bagel.
3. Layer smoked salmon, red onion, and tomato on one half.
4. Add capers if desired and place the other half of the bagel on top.
5. Serve immediately.

TIPS:
- Use a multigrain or whole-wheat bagel for added fiber.
- Add arugula for a peppery kick.

N.V.: Calories: 400, Fat: 20g, Carbs: 40g, Protein: 20g, Sugar: 5g

PEANUT BUTTER AND BANANA SMOOTHIE

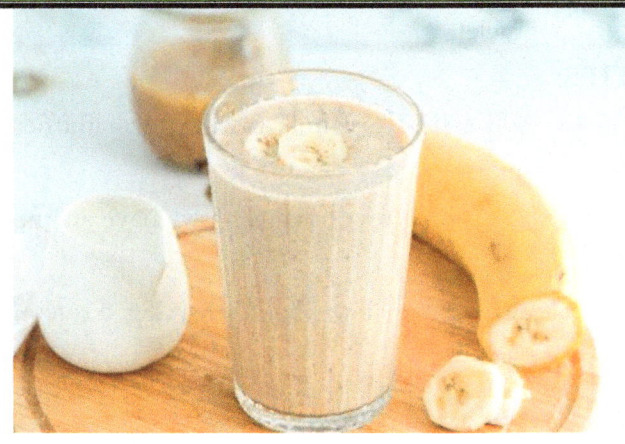

P.T.: 5 min.
C.T.: 0 min.
M.C: Blending
SERVINGS: 1
INGR:

- 1 ripe banana
- 1 Cup almond milk
- 2 Tbsp natural peanut butter
- 1 Tbsp honey
- 1/2 Tsp cinnamon
- Ice cubes

DIRECTIONS:

1. Combine banana, almond milk, peanut butter, honey, and cinnamon in a blender.
2. Add ice cubes to the blender.
3. Blend until smooth and creamy.
4. Pour into a glass and serve immediately.

TIPS:

- Add a scoop of protein powder for an extra protein boost.
- Use frozen banana slices for a thicker smoothie.

N.V.: Calories: 380, Fat: 18g, Carbs: 50g, Protein: 10g, Sugar: 25g

CHIA SEED PUDDING

P.T.: 5 min.
C.T.: 0 min. (Chill overnight)
M.C: None
SERVINGS: 2
INGR:

- 1/4 Cup chia seeds
- 1 Cup coconut milk
- 1 Tbsp maple syrup
- 1/2 Tsp vanilla extract
- Fresh berries for topping

DIRECTIONS:

1. In a bowl, mix chia seeds, coconut milk, maple syrup, and vanilla extract.
2. Stir well to combine and ensure no clumps.
3. Cover and refrigerate overnight or for at least 4 hours.
4. Serve topped with fresh berries.

TIPS:

- Stir once more after 30 minutes in the fridge to prevent clumping.
- Use almond milk for a lighter option.

N.V.: Calories: 250, Fat: 15g, Carbs: 25g, Protein: 6g, Sugar: 8g

2. BALANCED BREAKFAST MEALS

VEGGIE OMELET WITH WHOLE WHEAT TOAST

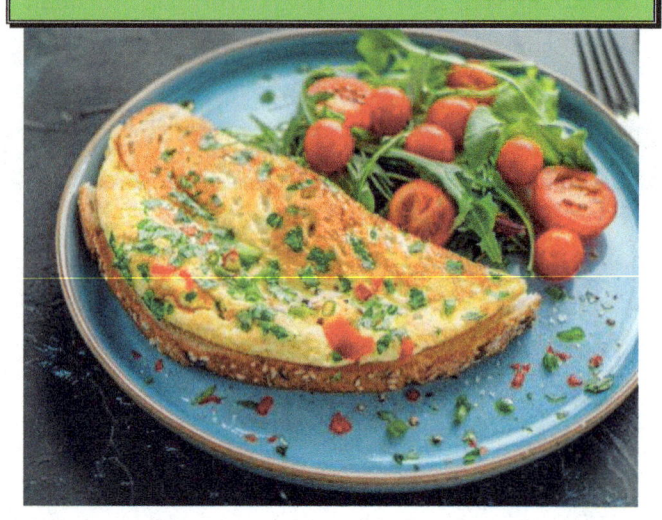

P.T.: 10 min.
C.T.: 10 min.
M.C: Stovetop
SERVINGS: 1
INGR:

- 3 large eggs
- 1/4 Cup bell peppers, diced
- 1/4 Cup spinach, chopped
- 1/4 Cup mushrooms, sliced
- 1/4 Cup onion, diced
- 1/4 Cup cheddar cheese, shredded
- 1 Tbsp olive oil
- Salt and pepper to taste
- 1 slice whole wheat bread

DIRECTIONS:

1. In a bowl, whisk the eggs with salt and pepper.
2. Heat olive oil in a skillet over medium heat.
3. Sauté bell peppers, spinach, mushrooms, and onions until soft.
4. Pour the eggs over the vegetables in the skillet.
5. Cook until the eggs are set, then sprinkle with cheese.
6. Fold the omelet and cook for an additional minute.
7. Toast the bread and serve alongside the omelet.

TIPS:

- Add a splash of milk to eggs for a fluffier omelet.
- Use any leftover veggies you have in the fridge.

N.V.: Calories: 500, Fat: 35g, Carbs: 28g, Protein: 25g, Sugar: 4g

QUINOA BREAKFAST BOWL

P.T.: 5 min.
C.T.: 15 min.
M.C: Stovetop
SERVINGS: 2
INGR:

- 1 Cup cooked quinoa
- 1/2 Cup almond milk
- 1 banana, sliced
- 1/4 Cup almonds, chopped
- 1 Tbsp chia seeds
- 1 Tbsp honey
- 1/2 Tsp cinnamon

DIRECTIONS:

1. In a saucepan, combine cooked quinoa and almond milk.
2. Heat over medium heat until warmed through.
3. Stir in banana slices, almonds, chia seeds, honey, and cinnamon.
4. Divide into bowls and serve immediately.

TIPS:

- Substitute almond milk with any milk of your choice.
- Add fresh berries for extra flavor and nutrients.

N.V.: Calories: 420, Fat: 14g, Carbs: 65g, Protein: 12g, Sugar: 18g

MEDITERRANEAN BREAKFAST WRAP

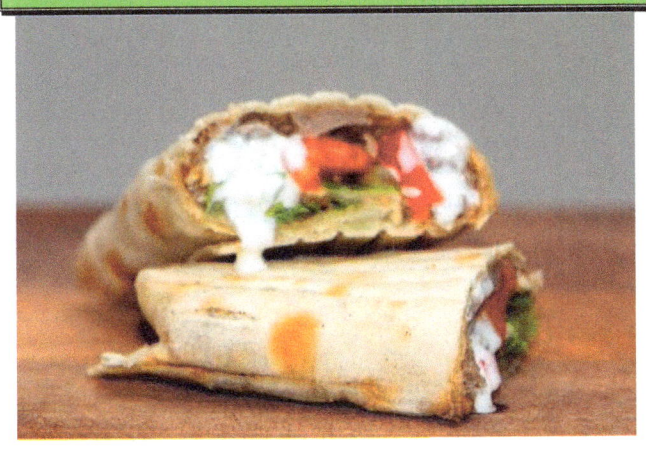

P.T.: 10 min.
C.T.: 5 min.
M.C: Stovetop
SERVINGS: 1
INGR:

- 1 whole wheat tortilla
- 2 large eggs
- 1/4 Cup feta cheese, crumbled
- 1/4 Cup cherry tomatoes, halved
- 1/4 Cup spinach, chopped
- 1 Tbsp olive oil
- Salt and pepper to taste

DIRECTIONS:

1. Heat olive oil in a skillet over medium heat.
2. Whisk eggs with salt and pepper, then pour into the skillet.
3. Scramble the eggs until fully cooked, then add feta, tomatoes, and spinach.
4. Place the egg mixture onto the tortilla and roll tightly.
5. Serve immediately, with additional fresh spinach if desired.

TIPS:

- Add olives for an authentic Mediterranean flavor.
- Use sun-dried tomatoes for a more intense taste.

N.V.: Calories: 450, Fat: 28g, Carbs: 35g, Protein: 21g, Sugar: 5g

SWEET POTATO AND BLACK BEAN HASH

P.T.: 10 min.
C.T.: 20 min.
M.C: Stovetop
SERVINGS: 2
INGR:

- 2 medium sweet potatoes, diced
- 1 can (15 oz) black beans, drained and rinsed
- 1/2 red onion, diced
- 1 red bell pepper, diced
- 2 cloves garlic, minced
- 2 Tbsp olive oil
- 1/2 Tsp cumin
- Salt and pepper to taste
- 2 eggs

DIRECTIONS:

1. Heat olive oil in a large skillet over medium heat.
2. Add sweet potatoes, onion, and bell pepper; sauté until tender.
3. Stir in garlic, black beans, cumin, salt, and pepper.
4. Cook until the sweet potatoes are fully cooked and beans are heated through.
5. In a separate pan, fry eggs to your preference.
6. Serve hash topped with a fried egg.

TIPS:

- Add avocado slices for creaminess.
- Top with fresh cilantro for a burst of flavor.

N.V.: Calories: 480, Fat: 20g, Carbs: 60g, Protein: 20g, Sugar: 10g

Cottage Cheese and Fruit Bowl

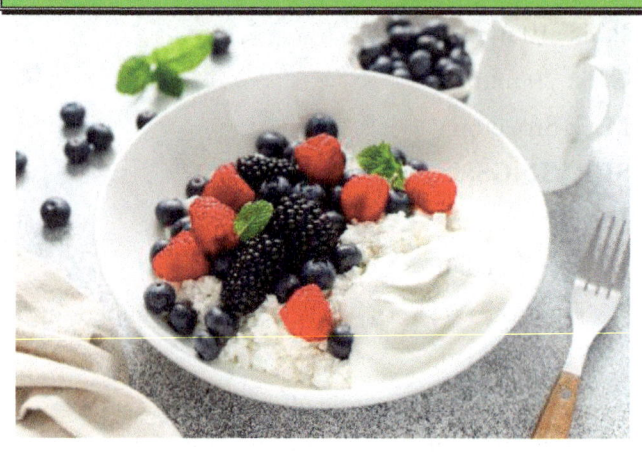

P.T.: 5 min.
C.T.: 0 min.
M.C: None
SERVINGS: 1
INGR:
- 1 Cup cottage cheese
- 1/2 Cup mixed berries (strawberries, blueberries, raspberries)
- 1 Tbsp honey
- 1/4 Cup granola
- 1/4 Cup walnuts, chopped

DIRECTIONS:
1. In a bowl, add cottage cheese.
2. Top with mixed berries, granola, and walnuts.
3. Drizzle with honey and serve immediately.

TIPS:
- Use Greek yogurt instead of cottage cheese for a different texture.
- Add chia seeds for extra fiber.

N.V.: Calories: 350, Fat: 18g, Carbs: 35g, Protein: 25g, Sugar: 15g

Egg and Avocado Sandwich

P.T.: 5 min.
C.T.: 10 min.
M.C: Stovetop
SERVINGS: 1
INGR:
- 2 slices whole grain bread
- 1 avocado, mashed
- 1 large egg
- 1 Tbsp butter
- Salt and pepper to taste
- 1 slice tomato
- 1 slice cheese (optional)

DIRECTIONS:
1. Toast the bread until golden brown.
2. Spread mashed avocado on one slice of bread.
3. Heat butter in a skillet over medium heat and fry the egg to your liking.
4. Place the egg on top of the avocado.
5. Add tomato slice and cheese if using, then top with the second slice of bread.
6. Serve immediately.

TIPS:
- Add bacon or turkey for extra protein.
- Season avocado with lime juice for a zesty flavor.

N.V.: Calories: 430, Fat: 28g, Carbs: 40g, Protein: 15g, Sugar: 5g

Overnight Oats with Almond Butter

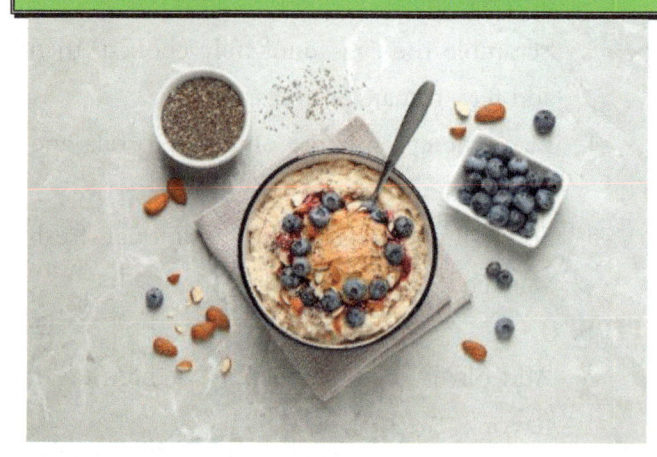

P.T.: 5 min.
C.T.: 0 min. (Chill overnight)
M.C: None
SERVINGS: 1

INGR:
- 1/2 Cup rolled oats
- 1/2 Cup almond milk
- 2 Tbsp almond butter
- 1 Tbsp chia seeds
- 1 Tbsp maple syrup
- 1/4 Cup blueberries

DIRECTIONS:
1. In a jar, combine oats, almond milk, almond butter, chia seeds, and maple syrup.
2. Stir well to combine.
3. Cover and refrigerate overnight.
4. Top with blueberries before serving.

TIPS:
- Add sliced banana for extra sweetness.
- Use peanut butter as a substitute for almond butter.

N.V.: Calories: 400, Fat: 18g, Carbs: 50g, Protein: 10g, Sugar: 12g3.

3. PREP-AHEAD IDEAS

BAKED OATMEAL CUPS

P.T.: 10 min
C.T.: 25 min
M.C: Baking
SERVINGS: 12 Cups
INGR:
- 2 Cups rolled oats
- 1/2 Cup almond milk
- 2 large eggs
- 1/4 Cup honey
- 1 Tsp vanilla extract
- 1/2 Tsp cinnamon
- 1/2 Tsp baking powder
- 1/4 Tsp salt
- 1/2 Cup blueberries
- 1/2 Cup diced apples
- 1/4 Cup chopped walnuts

DIRECTIONS:
1. Preheat oven to 350°F (175°C). Grease a muffin tin or line with paper liners.
2. In a large bowl, combine oats, almond milk, eggs, honey, vanilla extract, cinnamon, baking powder, and salt.
3. Fold in blueberries, apples, and walnuts.
4. Divide the mixture evenly among the muffin Cups.
5. Bake for 25 minutes or until golden and set.
6. Let cool before removing from the tin.

TIPS:
- Store in the fridge for up to a week.
- Freeze for longer storage and reheat in the microwave.

N.V.: Calories: 120 per Cup, Fat: 5g, Carbs: 16g, Protein: 3g, Sugar: 8g

OVERNIGHT CHIA SEED PUDDING

P.T.: 5 min
C.T.: 0 min. (Chill overnight)
M.C: None
SERVINGS: 4
INGR:
- 1/2 Cup chia seeds
- 2 Cups coconut milk
- 1 Tsp vanilla extract
- 1/4 Cup maple syrup
- Fresh fruit for topping (e.g., berries, mango)

DIRECTIONS:
1. In a large bowl, mix chia seeds, coconut milk, vanilla extract, and maple syrup.
2. Stir well to combine.
3. Cover and refrigerate overnight.
4. Stir before serving and top with fresh fruit.

TIPS:
- Stir after the first 30 minutes to prevent

clumping.
- Use any milk alternative for varied flavors.

N.V.: Calories: 200 per serving, Fat: 10g, Carbs: 26g, Protein: 4g, Sugar: 14g

Make-Ahead Breakfast Burritos

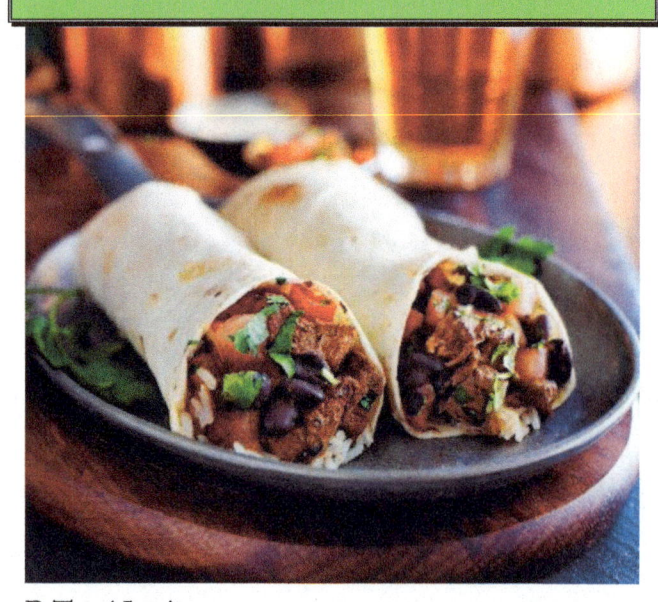

P.T.: 15 min
C.T.: 20 min
M.C: Stovetop
SERVINGS: 8
INGR:
- 8 whole wheat tortillas
- 8 large eggs
- 1 Cup black beans, drained and rinsed
- 1/2 Cup salsa
- 1 Cup shredded cheddar cheese
- 1 red bell pepper, diced
- 1 onion, diced
- 1 Tbsp olive oil
- Salt and pepper to taste

DIRECTIONS:
1. Heat olive oil in a skillet over medium heat.
2. Add onions and bell peppers; sauté until soft.
3. In a bowl, whisk eggs with salt and pepper. Pour into the skillet and scramble.
4. Stir in black beans and salsa until heated through.
5. Spoon the mixture onto each tortilla and top with cheese.
6. Roll tightly and wrap in foil. Store in the fridge or freezer.

TIPS:
- Reheat in the microwave for a quick breakfast.
- Use your favorite veggies to customize.

N.V.: Calories: 350 per burrito, Fat: 15g, Carbs: 36g, Protein: 18g, Sugar: 3g

Banana Bread Muffins

P.T.: 10 min
C.T.: 20 min
M.C: Baking
SERVINGS: 12 muffins
INGR:
- 3 ripe bananas, mashed
- 1/3 Cup melted butter
- 1/2 Cup sugar
- 1 large egg, beaten
- 1 Tsp vanilla extract
- 1 Tsp baking soda
- Pinch of salt
- 1 1/2 Cup s all-purpose flour

DIRECTIONS:
1. Preheat oven to 350°F (175°C). Line a muffin tin with paper liners.
2. In a bowl, mix mashed bananas, butter, sugar, egg, and vanilla.
3. Add baking soda and salt, then stir in flour until just combined.
4. Spoon the batter into the muffin tin.
5. Bake for 20 minutes or until a toothpick comes out clean.
6. Let cool on a wire rack.

TIPS:
- Add chocolate chips or nuts for variety.
- Store in an airtight container for up to a

week.

N.V.: Calories: 180 per muffin, Fat: 6g, Carbs: 30g, Protein: 3g, Sugar: 14g

SAVORY BREAKFAST QUICHE

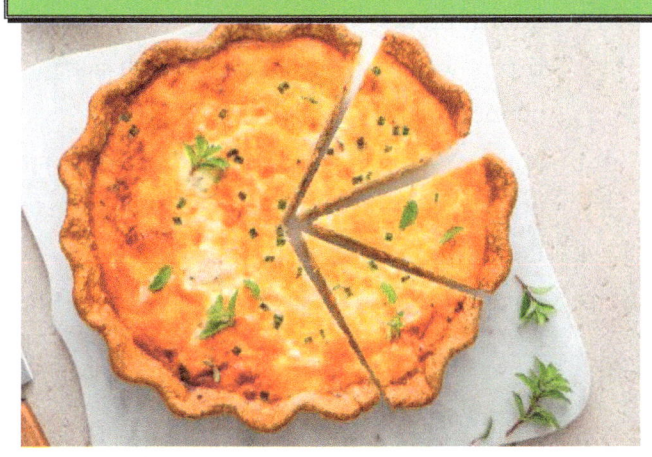

P.T.: 15 min
C.T.: 45 min
M.C: Baking
SERVINGS: 8
INGR:

- 1 pie crust (store-bought or homemade)
- 6 large eggs
- 1 Cup milk
- 1/2 Cup cheddar cheese, shredded
- 1 Cup spinach, chopped
- 1/2 Cup mushrooms, sliced
- 1/2 Cup ham, diced
- Salt and pepper to taste

DIRECTIONS:

1. Preheat oven to 375°F (190°C).
2. Roll out the pie crust and place it in a 9-inch pie dish.
3. In a bowl, whisk eggs and milk with salt and pepper.
4. Layer spinach, mushrooms, ham, and cheese in the pie crust.
5. Pour egg mixture over the ingredients.
6. Bake for 45 minutes or until the center is set.
7. Let cool before slicing.

TIPS:

- Customize with your favorite vegetables and proteins.
- Make ahead and reheat slices for a quick meal.

N.V.: Calories: 250 per slice, Fat: 15g, Carbs: 18g, Protein: 12g, Sugar: 2g

PROTEIN-PACKED BREAKFAST BARS

P.T.: 10 min
C.T.: 20 min
M.C: Baking
SERVINGS: 8 bars
INGR:

- 2 Cup s rolled oats
- 1/2 Cup almond butter
- 1/4 Cup honey
- 1/4 Cup protein powder
- 1/4 Cup almonds, chopped
- 1/4 Cup dark chocolate chips
- 1/2 Tsp vanilla extract

DIRECTIONS:

1. Preheat oven to 350°F (175°C). Line a baking dish with parchment paper.
2. In a bowl, mix oats, almond butter, honey, protein powder, almonds, chocolate chips, and vanilla.
3. Press the mixture into the baking dish.
4. Bake for 20 minutes or until golden.
5. Let cool before cutting into bars.

TIPS:

- Substitute almond butter with peanut butter if desired.
- Store in an airtight container for up to a week.

N.V.: Calories: 220 per bar, Fat: 10g, Carbs: 26g, Protein: 8g, Sugar: 12g

BREAKFAST EGG MUFFINS

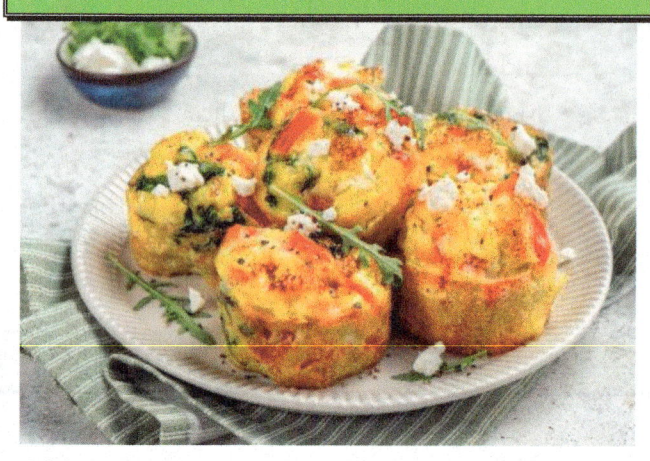

P.T.: 10 min
C.T.: 20 min
M.C: Baking
SERVINGS: 12 muffins
INGR:

- 8 large eggs
- 1/2 Cup milk
- 1/2 Cup cheddar cheese, shredded
- 1/2 Cup bell peppers, diced
- 1/2 Cup spinach, chopped
- 1/4 Cup onion, diced
- Salt and pepper to taste

DIRECTIONS:

1. Preheat oven to 375°F (190°C). Grease a muffin tin.
2. In a bowl, whisk eggs and milk with salt and pepper.
3. Stir in cheese, bell peppers, spinach, and onion.
4. Pour the mixture into the muffin tin.
5. Bake for 20 minutes or until the eggs are set.
6. Let cool before removing from the tin.

TIPS:

- Use muffin liners for easy cleanup.
- Customize with your favorite cheese and vegetables.

N.V.: Calories: 100 per muffin, Fat: 7g, Carbs: 2g, Protein: 8g, Sugar: 1g

CHAPTER 5: LUNCH SOLUTIONS
1. NUTRIENT-DENSE SALADS

KALE AND QUINOA SALAD WITH LEMON VINAIGRETTE

P.T.: 15 min
C.T.: 15 min
M.C: Stovetop (for quinoa)
SERVINGS: 4
INGR:

- 1 Cup quinoa
- 2 Cup s water
- 4 Cup s kale, chopped
- 1/2 Cup cherry tomatoes, halved
- 1/4 Cup red onion, thinly sliced
- 1/4 Cup sunflower seeds
- 1/4 Cup feta cheese, crumbled

Lemon Vinaigrette:

- 1/4 Cup olive oil
- 1/4 Cup lemon juice
- 1 Tsp Dijon mustard
- 1 Tsp honey
- Salt and pepper to taste

DIRECTIONS:

1. Rinse quinoa under cold water. In a saucepan, bring quinoa and water to a boil.
2. Reduce heat, cover, and simmer for 15 minutes until water is absorbed.
3. In a large bowl, combine kale, cooked quinoa, cherry tomatoes, red onion, sunflower seeds, and feta cheese.
4. In a small bowl, whisk together olive oil, lemon juice, Dijon mustard, honey, salt, and pepper.
5. Pour the vinaigrette over the salad and toss well to combine.

TIPS:

- Massage kale with a little olive oil to soften it before adding it to the salad.
- Add grilled chicken for extra protein.

N.V.: Calories: 320 per serving, Fat: 18g, Carbs: 30g, Protein: 10g, Sugar: 6g

SPINACH AND BERRY SALAD WITH POPPY SEED DRESSING

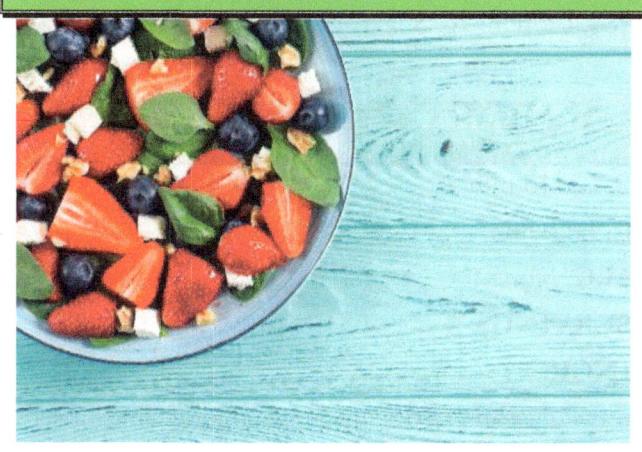

P.T.: 10 min
C.T.: 0 min
M.C: None
SERVINGS: 4
INGR:

- 6 Cup s baby spinach
- 1 Cup strawberries, sliced
- 1/2 Cup blueberries
- 1/4 Cup almonds, sliced
- 1/4 Cup goat cheese, crumbled

Poppy Seed Dressing:

- 1/4 Cup olive oil
- 2 Tbsp apple cider vinegar
- 1 Tbsp honey
- 1 Tsp poppy seeds
- Salt and pepper to taste

DIRECTIONS:

1. In a large bowl, combine spinach, strawberries, blueberries, almonds, and goat cheese.
2. In a small bowl, whisk together olive oil, apple cider vinegar, honey, poppy seeds,

salt, and pepper.
3. Drizzle the dressing over the salad and toss gently to combine.

TIPS:
- Substitute goat cheese with feta cheese if desired.
- Add avocado slices for extra creaminess.

N.V.: Calories: 280 per serving, Fat: 20g, Carbs: 18g, Protein: 7g, Sugar: 11g

MEDITERRANEAN CHICKPEA SALAD

P.T.: 15 min
C.T.: 0 min
M.C: None
SERVINGS: 4
INGR:
- 1 can (15 oz) chickpeas, drained and rinsed
- 1 Cup cucumber, diced
- 1 Cup cherry tomatoes, halved
- 1/4 Cup red onion, diced
- 1/4 Cup Kalamata olives, sliced
- 1/4 Cup feta cheese, crumbled
- 2 Tbsp fresh parsley, chopped

Dressing:
- 3 Tbsp olive oil
- 1 Tbsp red wine vinegar
- 1 Tsp dried oregano
- Salt and pepper to taste

DIRECTIONS:
1. In a large bowl, combine chickpeas, cucumber, cherry tomatoes, red onion, olives, feta cheese, and parsley.
2. In a small bowl, whisk together olive oil, red wine vinegar, oregano, salt, and pepper.
3. Pour the dressing over the salad and toss to coat evenly.

TIPS:
- Let the salad sit for at least 30 minutes to allow flavors to meld.
- Add a squeeze of lemon juice for extra brightness.

N.V.: Calories: 320 per serving, Fat: 18g, Carbs: 30g, Protein: 10g, Sugar: 3g

GRILLED CHICKEN CAESAR SALAD

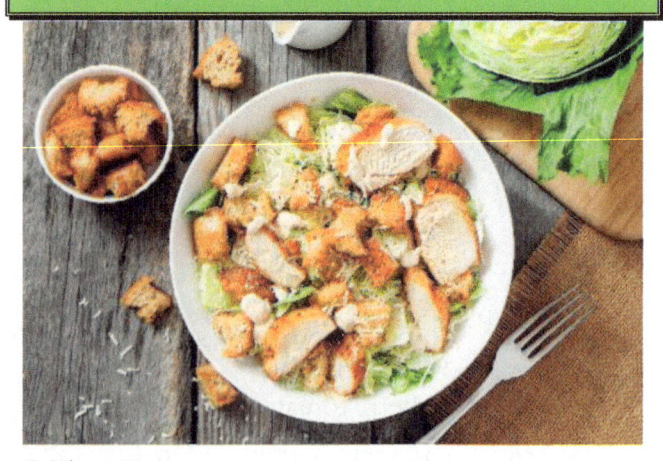

P.T.: 10 min
C.T.: 10 min
M.C: Grill/Stovetop
SERVINGS: 4
INGR:
- 2 boneless, skinless chicken breasts
- 6 Cup s Romaine lettuce, chopped
- 1/2 Cup Parmesan cheese, shaved
- 1 Cup croutons

Caesar Dressing:
- 1/4 Cup olive oil
- 2 Tbsp lemon juice
- 1 Tsp Dijon mustard
- 1 clove garlic, minced
- Salt and pepper to taste

DIRECTIONS:
1. Season chicken breasts with salt and pepper. Grill or cook on a stovetop until fully cooked, about 5 minutes per side. Let rest, then slice.
2. In a large bowl, combine Romaine lettuce, Parmesan cheese, and croutons.
3. In a small bowl, whisk together olive oil, lemon juice, Dijon mustard, garlic, salt, and pepper.

4. Drizzle dressing over the salad and toss to combine.
   5. Top with sliced chicken and serve.

TIPS:
- Use rotisserie chicken for a quicker preparation.
- Add anchovies for an authentic Caesar flavor.

N.V.: Calories: 400 per serving, Fat: 25g, Carbs: 20g, Protein: 25g, Sugar: 2g

ASIAN SESAME SALAD WITH GRILLED TOFU

P.T.: 15 min
C.T.: 10 min
M.C: Grill/Stovetop
SERVINGS: 4
INGR:
- 1 block (14 oz) firm tofu, pressed and sliced
- 4 Cup s mixed greens
- 1 Cup red cabbage, shredded
- 1/2 Cup carrots, julienned
- 1/4 Cup green onions, chopped
- 2 Tbsp sesame seeds, toasted

Sesame Dressing:
- 3 Tbsp soy sauce
- 2 Tbsp rice vinegar
- 1 Tbsp sesame oil
- 1 Tbsp honey
- 1 Tsp ginger, grated

DIRECTIONS:
1. Grill or pan-fry tofu slices until golden brown, about 5 minutes per side.
2. In a large bowl, combine mixed greens, cabbage, carrots, and green onions.
3. In a small bowl, whisk together soy sauce, rice vinegar, sesame oil, honey, and ginger.
4. Add tofu to the salad and drizzle with dressing. Toss to combine.
5. Sprinkle with sesame seeds before serving.

TIPS:
- Add edamame for extra protein.
- Use chicken or shrimp instead of tofu for a variation.

N.V.: Calories: 350 per serving, Fat: 22g, Carbs: 22g, Protein: 18g, Sugar: 9g

ROASTED VEGETABLE AND FARRO SALAD

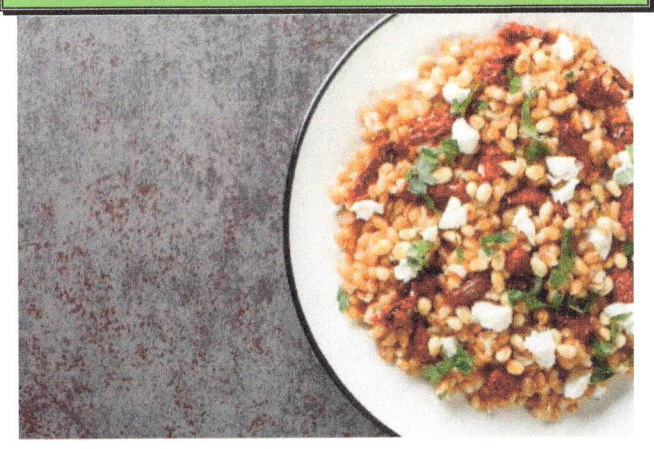

P.T.: 15 min
C.T.: 25 min
M.C: Roasting/Stovetop
SERVINGS: 4
INGR:
- 1 Cup farro
- 2 Cup s water
- 1 zucchini, diced
- 1 red bell pepper, diced
- 1 Cup cherry tomatoes, halved
- 1/4 Cup red onion, sliced
- 2 Tbsp olive oil
- Salt and pepper to taste
- 1/4 Cup feta cheese, crumbled

Dressing:
- 3 Tbsp olive oil
- 1 Tbsp balsamic vinegar
- 1 Tsp honey
- Salt and pepper to taste

DIRECTIONS:
1. Preheat oven to 400°F (204°C). Toss zucchini, bell pepper, cherry tomatoes, and

onion with olive oil, salt, and pepper. Roast for 20 minutes.

2. Meanwhile, rinse farro and cook in boiling water for 25 minutes or until tender. Drain and let cool.
3. In a large bowl, combine roasted vegetables, farro, and feta cheese.
4. In a small bowl, whisk together olive oil, balsamic vinegar, honey, salt, and pepper.
5. Pour dressing over the salad and toss to combine.

TIPS:
- Serve warm or cold, depending on preference.
- Substitute quinoa for farro if desired.

N.V.: Calories: 340 per serving, Fat: 15g, Carbs: 42g, Protein: 10g, Sugar: 8g

BEET AND ARUGULA SALAD WITH GOAT CHEESE

P.T.: 10 min
C.T.: 45 min (for roasting beets)
M.C: Roasting
SERVINGS: 4
INGR:
- 4 medium beets
- 6 Cup s arugula
- 1/4 Cup walnuts, toasted
- 1/4 Cup goat cheese, crumbled

Dressing:
- 3 Tbsp olive oil
- 1 Tbsp balsamic vinegar
- 1 Tsp Dijon mustard
- Salt and pepper to taste

DIRECTIONS:
1. Preheat oven to 400°F (204°C). Wrap beets in foil and roast for 45 minutes or until tender. Let cool, then peel and slice.
2. In a large bowl, combine arugula, roasted beets, walnuts, and goat cheese.
3. In a small bowl, whisk together olive oil, balsamic vinegar, Dijon mustard, salt, and pepper.
4. Drizzle dressing over the salad and toss gently to combine.

TIPS:
- Use pre-cooked beets to save time.
- Add orange segments for a sweet contrast.

N.V.: Calories: 300 per serving, Fat: 20g, Carbs: 24g, Protein: 6g, Sugar: 14g

2. HEARTY SOUPS AND STEWS

CREAMY BUTTERNUT SQUASH SOUP

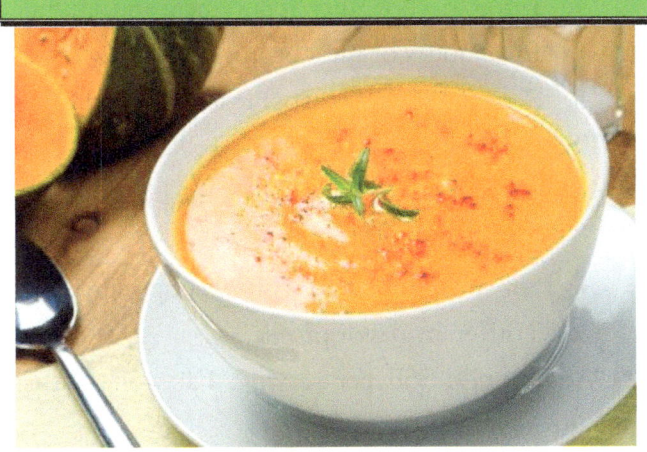

P.T.: 15 min
C.T.: 45 min
M.C: Stovetop
SERVINGS: 6
INGR:

- 2 lbs butternut squash, peeled and cubed
- 1 onion, chopped
- 2 carrots, sliced
- 2 cloves garlic, minced
- 4 Cup s vegetable broth
- 1 Cup coconut milk
- 1 Tbsp olive oil
- 1 Tsp ground cumin
- Salt and pepper to taste
- Fresh cilantro for garnish

DIRECTIONS:

1. Heat olive oil in a large pot over medium heat. Add onion, carrots, and garlic. Sauté until onions are translucent.
2. Add butternut squash, cumin, salt, and pepper. Stir to combine.
3. Pour in vegetable broth and bring to a boil. Reduce heat and simmer for 30 minutes or until squash is tender.
4. Using an immersion blender, puree the soup until smooth.
5. Stir in coconut milk and heat through.
6. Serve hot, garnished with fresh cilantro.

TIPS:

- For a spicier version, add a pinch of cayenne pepper.
- Use an immersion blender directly in the pot for easier cleanup.

N.V.: Calories: 200 per serving, Fat: 10g, Carbs: 28g, Protein: 3g, Sugar: 8g

CLASSIC CHICKEN NOODLE SOUP

P.T.: 10 min
C.T.: 30 min
M.C: Stovetop
SERVINGS: 6
INGR:

- 2 lbs chicken breast, diced
- 2 carrots, sliced
- 2 celery stalks, sliced
- 1 onion, chopped
- 3 cloves garlic, minced
- 6 Cup s chicken broth
- 1 Cup egg noodles
- 2 Tbsp olive oil
- 1 Tsp dried thyme
- Salt and pepper to taste
- Fresh parsley for garnish

DIRECTIONS:

1. Heat olive oil in a large pot over medium heat. Add chicken and cook until browned. Remove and set aside.
2. In the same pot, add onion, carrots, celery, and garlic. Sauté until vegetables are tender.
3. Return chicken to the pot. Add chicken broth, thyme, salt, and pepper. Bring to a boil.
4. Add egg noodles and simmer for 10 minutes or until noodles are cooked.
5. Serve hot, garnished with fresh parsley.

TIPS:
- Use rotisserie chicken for a quicker version.
- Add a squeeze of lemon juice for added brightness.

N.V.: Calories: 250 per serving, Fat: 10g, Carbs: 18g, Protein: 25g, Sugar: 2g

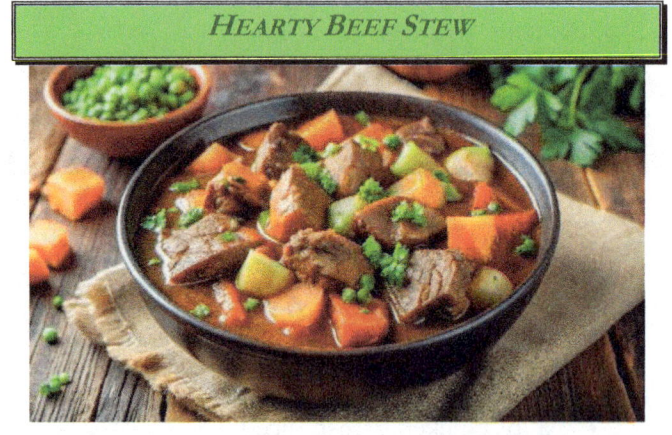

Hearty Beef Stew

P.T.: 20 min
C.T.: 2 hr
M.C: Stovetop
SERVINGS: 6
INGR:
- 2 lbs beef stew meat, cubed
- 3 carrots, sliced
- 3 potatoes, cubed
- 1 onion, chopped
- 3 cloves garlic, minced
- 4 Cup s beef broth
- 2 Tbsp tomato paste
- 2 Tbsp olive oil
- 1 Tsp dried rosemary
- 1 Tsp dried thyme
- Salt and pepper to taste

DIRECTIONS:
1. Heat olive oil in a large pot over medium heat. Add beef and cook until browned on all sides. Remove and set aside.
2. In the same pot, add onion, carrots, potatoes, and garlic. Sauté until vegetables begin to soften.
3. Return beef to the pot. Add beef broth, tomato paste, rosemary, thyme, salt, and pepper. Stir to combine.
4. Bring to a boil, then reduce heat and simmer for 2 hours or until beef is tender.
5. Serve hot, with crusty bread if desired.

TIPS:
- For a thicker stew, mash some potatoes and stir them back into the stew.
- Substitute potatoes with sweet potatoes for a different flavor profile.

N.V.: Calories: 350 per serving, Fat: 15g, Carbs: 30g, Protein: 25g, Sugar: 4g

Lentil and Spinach Soup

P.T.: 10 min
C.T.: 40 min
M.C: Stovetop
SERVINGS: 6
INGR:
- 1 Cup lentils, rinsed
- 1 onion, chopped
- 2 carrots, diced
- 2 celery stalks, diced
- 3 cloves garlic, minced
- 6 Cup s vegetable broth
- 2 Cup s spinach, chopped
- 2 Tbsp olive oil
- 1 Tsp ground cumin
- Salt and pepper to taste

DIRECTIONS:
1. Heat olive oil in a large pot over medium heat. Add onion, carrots, celery, and garlic. Sauté until vegetables are tender.
2. Stir in lentils, cumin, salt, and pepper.
3. Add vegetable broth and bring to a boil. Reduce heat and simmer for 30 minutes or until lentils are tender.
4. Stir in spinach and cook until wilted.
5. Serve hot, with a drizzle of olive oil if desired.

TIPS:
- Add diced tomatoes for extra flavor.
- Top with a dollop of Greek yogurt for creaminess.

N.V.: Calories: 220 per serving, Fat: 8g, Carbs: 30g, Protein: 12g, Sugar: 4g

MINESTRONE SOUP

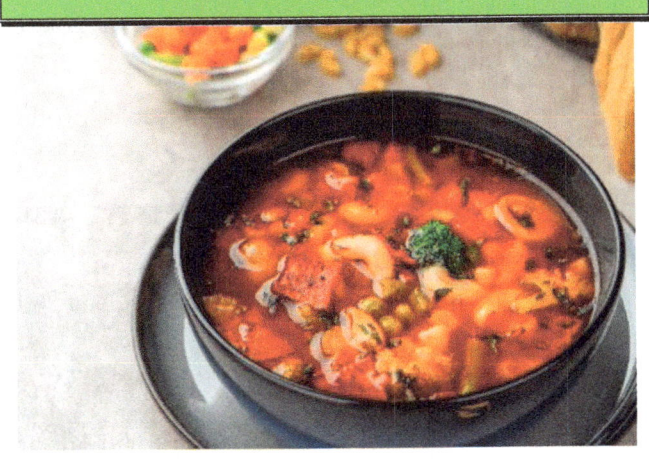

P.T.: 15 min
C.T.: 40 min
M.C: Stovetop
SERVINGS: 6
INGR:
- 1 onion, chopped
- 2 carrots, diced
- 2 celery stalks, diced
- 2 cloves garlic, minced
- 1 zucchini, diced
- 1 can (15 oz) kidney beans, drained and rinsed
- 1 can (15 oz) diced tomatoes
- 4 Cups vegetable broth
- 1 Cup small pasta
- 1 Tsp dried oregano
- Salt and pepper to taste
- Fresh basil for garnish

DIRECTIONS:
1. Heat olive oil in a large pot over medium heat. Add onion, carrots, celery, and garlic. Sauté until vegetables are tender.
2. Stir in zucchini, kidney beans, diced tomatoes, oregano, salt, and pepper.
3. Add vegetable broth and bring to a boil. Reduce heat and simmer for 20 minutes.
4. Stir in pasta and cook for an additional 10 minutes or until pasta is al dente.
5. Serve hot, garnished with fresh basil.

TIPS:
- Use any small pasta shape you prefer.
- Add Parmesan cheese for extra flavor.

N.V.: Calories: 290 per serving, Fat: 6g, Carbs: 50g, Protein: 12g, Sugar: 7g

MOROCCAN CHICKPEA STEW

P.T.: 10 min
C.T.: 30 min
M.C: Stovetop
SERVINGS: 6
INGR:
- 1 onion, chopped
- 2 carrots, diced
- 2 cloves garlic, minced
- 1 can (15 oz) chickpeas, drained and rinsed
- 1 can (15 oz) diced tomatoes
- 2 Cups vegetable broth
- 1 Tsp ground cumin
- 1 Tsp ground coriander
- 1/2 Tsp cinnamon
- Salt and pepper to taste
- 1/4 Cup fresh cilantro, chopped

DIRECTIONS:
1. Heat olive oil in a large pot over medium heat. Add onion, carrots, and garlic. Sauté until vegetables are tender.
2. Stir in chickpeas, diced tomatoes, cumin, coriander, cinnamon, salt, and pepper.
3. Add vegetable broth and bring to a boil. Reduce heat and simmer for 20 minutes.
4. Serve hot, garnished with fresh cilantro.

TIPS:
- Add raisins for a touch of sweetness.
- Serve with couscous or rice for a complete meal.

N.V.: Calories: 240 per serving, Fat: 5g, Carbs: 40g, Protein: 10g, Sugar: 8g

THAI COCONUT CURRY SOUP

P.T.: 10 min
C.T.: 20 min
M.C: Stovetop
SERVINGS: 6
INGR:
- 1 Tbsp olive oil
- 1 onion, sliced
- 1 red bell pepper, sliced
- 3 cloves garlic, minced
- 1 Tbsp ginger, grated
- 2 Cup s coconut milk
- 2 Cup s vegetable broth
- 1 Tbsp red curry paste
- 1 Cup tofu, cubed
- 1 Cup mushrooms, sliced
- 1 Cup snow peas
- Salt to taste
- Lime wedges and fresh cilantro for garnish

DIRECTIONS:
1. Heat olive oil in a large pot over medium heat. Add onion, bell pepper, garlic, and ginger. Sauté until fragrant.
2. Stir in red curry paste and cook for 1 minute.
3. Add coconut milk and vegetable broth, bring to a simmer.
4. Add tofu, mushrooms, and snow peas. Cook for 10 minutes.
5. Serve hot, garnished with lime wedges and fresh cilantro.

TIPS:
- Adjust the curry paste to taste for more or less heat.
- Add cooked rice noodles for a heartier meal.

N.V.: Calories: 320 per serving, Fat: 22g, Carbs: 24g, Protein: 10g, Sugar: 4g

3. PORTABLE LUNCHES

TURKEY AND AVOCADO WRAP

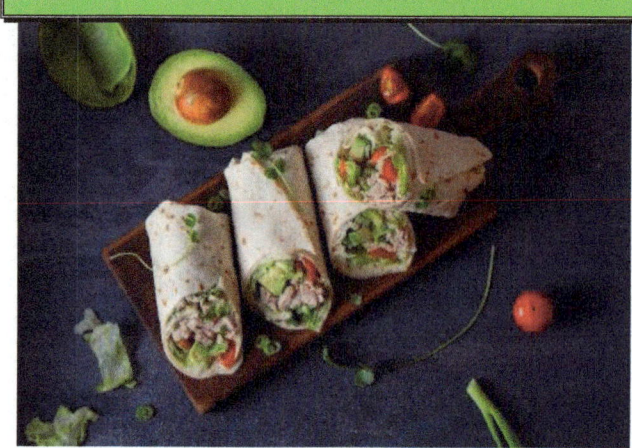

P.T.: 10 min
C.T.: 0 min
M.C: None
SERVINGS: 1
INGR:
- 1 whole wheat tortilla
- 4 oz sliced turkey breast
- 1/2 avocado, sliced
- 1/4 Cup baby spinach
- 1/4 Cup shredded carrots
- 2 Tbsp hummus
- Salt and pepper to taste

DIRECTIONS:
1. Spread hummus evenly over the tortilla.
2. Layer turkey, avocado, spinach, and carrots on top of the hummus.
3. Season with salt and pepper.
4. Roll the tortilla tightly into a wrap.
5. Slice in half and serve, or wrap in foil for

easy transport.

TIPS:
- Add a squeeze of lemon juice to prevent the avocado from browning.
- Substitute turkey with chicken or roasted vegetables for variety.

N.V.: Calories: 420, Fat: 20g, Carbs: 40g, Protein: 24g, Sugar: 4g

QUINOA AND BLACK BEAN SALAD

P.T.: 15 min
C.T.: 15 min
M.C: Stovetop
SERVINGS: 4
INGR:
- 1 Cup quinoa
- 2 Cup s water
- 1 can (15 oz) black beans, drained and rinsed
- 1 Cup cherry tomatoes, halved
- 1/2 Cup corn kernels (fresh or frozen)
- 1/4 Cup red onion, diced
- 1/4 Cup cilantro, chopped
- 2 Tbsp olive oil
- 2 Tbsp lime juice
- 1 Tsp cumin
- Salt and pepper to taste

DIRECTIONS:
1. Rinse quinoa under cold water. In a saucepan, bring quinoa and water to a boil.
2. Reduce heat, cover, and simmer for 15 minutes until water is absorbed. Let cool.
3. In a large bowl, combine cooked quinoa, black beans, cherry tomatoes, corn, red onion, and cilantro.
4. In a small bowl, whisk together olive oil, lime juice, cumin, salt, and pepper.
5. Pour dressing over the salad and toss to combine.

TIPS:
- Serve chilled or at room temperature.
- Add diced avocado for extra creaminess.

N.V.: Calories: 360 per serving, Fat: 12g, Carbs: 52g, Protein: 12g, Sugar: 3g

GREEK PASTA SALAD

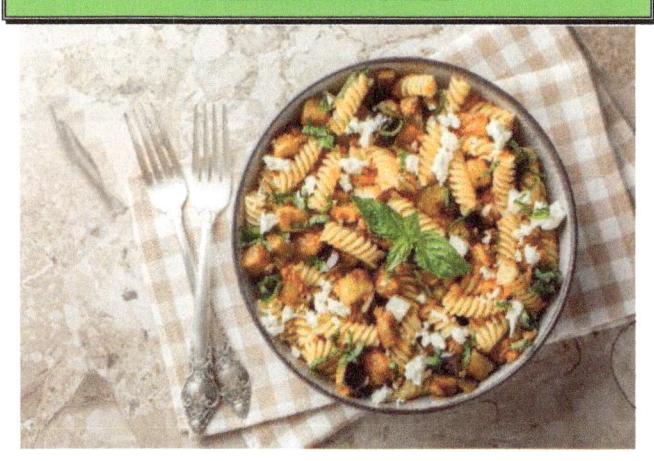

P.T.: 10 min
C.T.: 10 min
M.C: Stovetop
SERVINGS: 4
INGR:
- 8 oz whole wheat pasta
- 1 Cup cherry tomatoes, halved
- 1/2 Cup cucumber, diced
- 1/4 Cup Kalamata olives, sliced
- 1/4 Cup red onion, sliced
- 1/2 Cup feta cheese, crumbled
- 1/4 Cup olive oil
- 2 Tbsp red wine vinegar
- 1 Tsp dried oregano
- Salt and pepper to taste

DIRECTIONS:
1. Cook pasta according to package instructions. Drain and let cool.
2. In a large bowl, combine pasta, cherry tomatoes, cucumber, olives, red onion, and feta cheese.
3. In a small bowl, whisk together olive oil, red wine vinegar, oregano, salt, and pepper.

4. Pour dressing over the salad and toss to combine.

TIPS:
- Use gluten-free pasta if desired.
- Add grilled chicken for extra protein.

N.V.: Calories: 380 per serving, Fat: 18g, Carbs: 46g, Protein: 12g, Sugar: 4g

Caprese Sandwich

P.T.: 10 min
C.T.: 0 min
M.C: None
SERVINGS: 1
INGR:
- 1 ciabatta roll
- 2 oz fresh mozzarella, sliced
- 1 tomato, sliced
- 1/4 Cup fresh basil leaves
- 1 Tbsp balsamic glaze
- 1 Tbsp olive oil
- Salt and pepper to taste

DIRECTIONS:
1. Slice the ciabatta roll in half.
2. Drizzle olive oil on the inside of both halves.
3. Layer mozzarella, tomato, and basil leaves on the bottom half.
4. Drizzle with balsamic glaze and season with salt and pepper.
5. Place the top half of the roll over the filling and press gently.
6. Wrap in foil for transport.

TIPS:
- Toast the ciabatta for added crunch.
- Add a slice of prosciutto for a savory twist.

N.V.: Calories: 450, Fat: 22g, Carbs: 44g, Protein: 16g, Sugar: 5g

Asian Chicken Lettuce Wraps

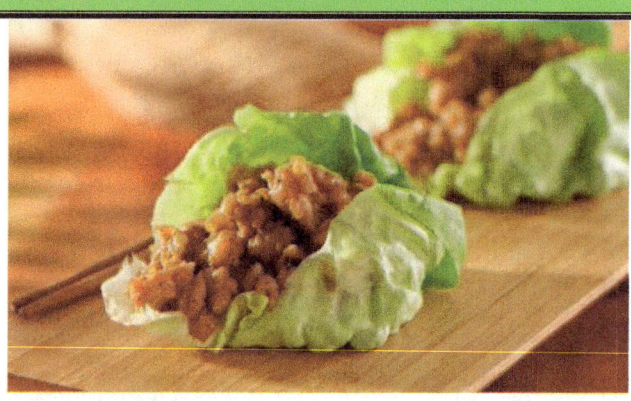

P.T.: 15 min
C.T.: 10 min
M.C: Stovetop
SERVINGS: 4
INGR:
- 1 lb ground chicken
- 1/2 Cup water chestnuts, chopped
- 1/4 Cup green onions, sliced
- 1/4 Cup hoisin sauce
- 1 Tbsp soy sauce
- 1 Tbsp sesame oil
- 1 Tsp ginger, minced
- 1 clove garlic, minced
- 8 large lettuce leaves (e.g., butter or iceberg)
- Sesame seeds for garnish

DIRECTIONS:
1. Heat sesame oil in a skillet over medium heat. Add garlic and ginger, sauté until fragrant.
2. Add ground chicken and cook until browned.
3. Stir in water chestnuts, green onions, hoisin sauce, and soy sauce. Cook for 2-3 minutes.
4. Spoon chicken mixture onto lettuce leaves.
5. Garnish with sesame seeds and serve.

TIPS:
- Use ground turkey or beef as an alternative.
- Add sriracha for a spicy kick.

N.V.: Calories: 320 per serving, Fat: 18g, Carbs: 14g, Protein: 26g, Sugar: 7g

ROASTED VEGETABLE AND HUMMUS WRAP

P.T.: 10 min
C.T.: 20 min
M.C: Roasting
SERVINGS: 4
INGR:
- 1 zucchini, sliced
- 1 red bell pepper, sliced
- 1 onion, sliced
- 1 Cup mushrooms, sliced
- 2 Tbsp olive oil
- Salt and pepper to taste
- 1 Cup hummus
- 4 whole wheat tortillas
- 1/4 Cup feta cheese, crumbled

DIRECTIONS:
1. Preheat oven to 400°F (204°C). Toss vegetables with olive oil, salt, and pepper.
2. Spread vegetables on a baking sheet and roast for 20 minutes or until tender.
3. Spread hummus on each tortilla.
4. Divide roasted vegetables among the tortillas and sprinkle with feta cheese.
5. Roll each tortilla tightly into a wrap and serve.

TIPS:
- Add arugula for a peppery flavor.
- Use different seasonal vegetables for variety.

N.V.: Calories: 360 per serving, Fat: 18g, Carbs: 42g, Protein: 10g, Sugar: 5g

TUNA AND WHITE BEAN SALAD

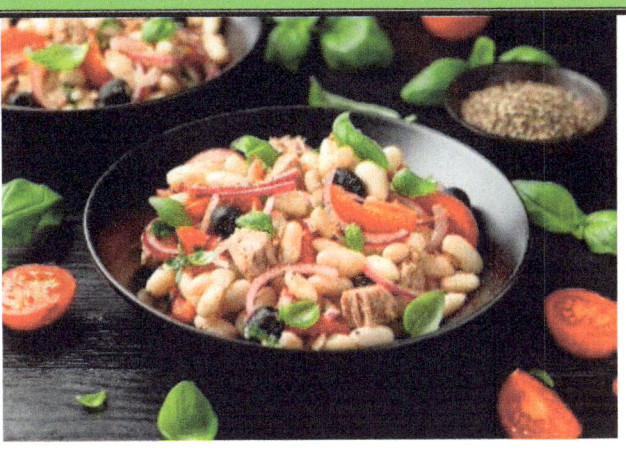

P.T.: 10 min
C.T.: 0 min
M.C: None
SERVINGS: 4
INGR:
- 2 cans (5 oz each) tuna, drained
- 1 can (15 oz) cannellini beans, drained and rinsed
- 1/2 Cup cherry tomatoes, halved
- 1/4 Cup red onion, diced
- 1/4 Cup parsley, chopped
- 2 Tbsp olive oil
- 2 Tbsp lemon juice
- Salt and pepper to taste

DIRECTIONS:
1. In a large bowl, combine tuna, cannellini beans, cherry tomatoes, red onion, and parsley.
2. In a small bowl, whisk together olive oil, lemon juice, salt, and pepper.
3. Pour dressing over the salad and toss gently to combine.

TIPS:
- Serve over mixed greens for added volume.
- Add capers for a briny flavor.

N.V.: Calories: 300 per serving, Fat: 12g, Carbs: 20g, Protein: 26g, Sugar: 1g

CHAPTER 6: DINNER DELIGHTS

1. LEAN PROTEINS

GRILLED LEMON HERB CHICKEN

P.T.: 10 min
C.T.: 20 min
M.C: Grilling
SERVINGS: 4
INGR:

- 4 boneless, skinless chicken breasts
- 1/4 Cup olive oil
- 2 Tbsp lemon juice
- 2 cloves garlic, minced
- 1 Tsp dried oregano
- 1 Tsp dried thyme
- Salt and pepper to taste
- Lemon slices for garnish

DIRECTIONS:

1. In a bowl, whisk together olive oil, lemon juice, garlic, oregano, thyme, salt, and pepper.
2. Place chicken breasts in a resealable bag and pour marinade over them. Seal and refrigerate for at least 30 minutes.
3. Preheat grill to medium-high heat.
4. Remove chicken from marinade and grill for 6-7 minutes on each side or until fully cooked.
5. Serve hot, garnished with lemon slices.

TIPS:

- Let chicken rest for 5 minutes before slicing to retain juices.
- Add rosemary for additional flavor.

N.V.: Calories: 300 per serving, Fat: 15g, Carbs: 2g, Protein: 36g, Sugar: 0g

BAKED SALMON WITH DILL AND LEMON

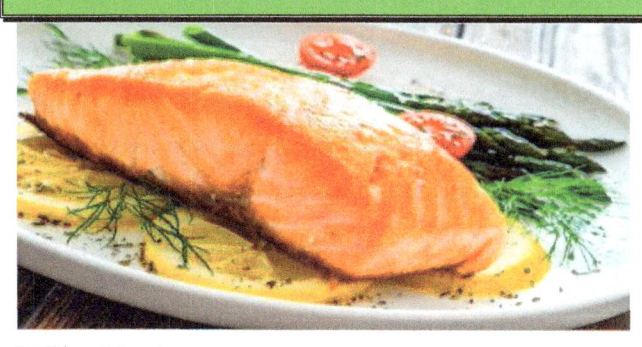

P.T.: 10 min
C.T.: 20 min
M.C: Baking
SERVINGS: 4
INGR:

- 4 salmon fillets
- 2 Tbsp olive oil
- 1 lemon, sliced
- 1 Tbsp fresh dill, chopped
- Salt and pepper to taste

DIRECTIONS:

1. Preheat oven to 400°F (204°C).
2. Place salmon fillets on a baking sheet lined with parchment paper.
3. Drizzle with olive oil and season with salt and pepper.
4. Top each fillet with lemon slices and sprinkle with dill.
5. Bake for 15-20 minutes or until salmon flakes easily with a fork.

TIPS:

- Use parchment paper for easy cleanup.
- Serve with steamed asparagus or green beans.

N.V.: Calories: 350 per serving, Fat: 22g, Carbs: 1g, Protein: 36g, Sugar: 0g

Turkey Stuffed Bell Peppers

P.T.: 15 min
C.T.: 30 min
M.C: Baking
SERVINGS: 4
INGR:

- 4 large bell peppers, halved and seeded
- 1 lb ground turkey
- 1 Cup cooked quinoa
- 1 can (15 oz) diced tomatoes, drained
- 1 onion, diced
- 2 cloves garlic, minced
- 1 Tsp Italian seasoning
- 1 Cup shredded mozzarella cheese
- Salt and pepper to taste

DIRECTIONS:

1. Preheat oven to 375°F (190°C).
2. In a skillet, cook ground turkey with onion and garlic until browned.
3. Stir in quinoa, diced tomatoes, Italian seasoning, salt, and pepper.
4. Spoon turkey mixture into each bell pepper half.
5. Place stuffed peppers in a baking dish and top with mozzarella cheese.
6. Bake for 30 minutes or until peppers are tender.

TIPS:

- Use different colored peppers for a vibrant presentation.
- Substitute quinoa with brown rice if desired.

N.V.: Calories: 400 per serving, Fat: 15g, Carbs: 35g, Protein: 35g, Sugar: 5g

Herb-Crusted Pork Tenderloin

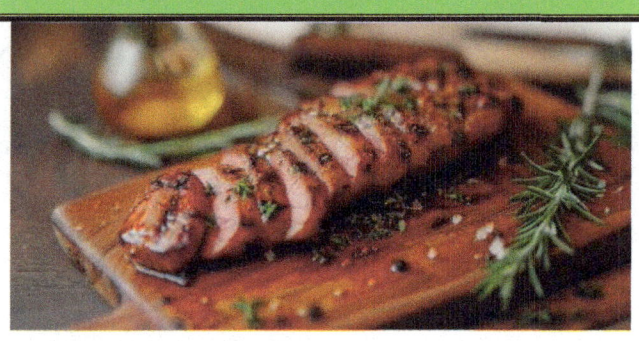

P.T.: 10 min
C.T.: 30 min
M.C: Roasting
SERVINGS: 4
INGR:

- 1.5 lbs pork tenderloin
- 2 Tbsp olive oil
- 2 cloves garlic, minced
- 1 Tbsp fresh rosemary, chopped
- 1 Tbsp fresh thyme, chopped
- Salt and pepper to taste

DIRECTIONS:

1. Preheat oven to 425°F (220°C).
2. In a bowl, mix olive oil, garlic, rosemary, thyme, salt, and pepper.
3. Rub mixture evenly over pork tenderloin.
4. Place tenderloin in a roasting pan and roast for 25-30 minutes or until internal temperature reaches 145°F (63°C).
5. Let rest for 5 minutes before slicing.

TIPS:

- Serve with roasted vegetables for a complete meal.
- Use a meat thermometer for precise cooking.

N.V.: Calories: 300 per serving, Fat: 15g, Carbs: 1g, Protein: 38g, Sugar: 0g

GARLIC SHRIMP STIR-FRY

P.T.: 10 min
C.T.: 10 min
M.C: Stovetop
SERVINGS: 4
INGR:

- 1 lb large shrimp, peeled and deveined
- 2 Tbsp olive oil
- 3 cloves garlic, minced
- 1 red bell pepper, sliced
- 1 Cup snow peas
- 2 Tbsp soy sauce
- 1 Tsp ginger, grated
- Salt and pepper to taste

DIRECTIONS:

1. Heat olive oil in a large skillet over medium heat.
2. Add garlic and ginger, sauté until fragrant.
3. Add shrimp and cook for 2-3 minutes on each side until pink.
4. Stir in bell pepper and snow peas, cook for 3-4 minutes.
5. Add soy sauce and toss to coat.
6. Serve hot, over brown rice if desired.

TIPS:

- Substitute shrimp with scallops or chicken.
- Add a splash of sesame oil for extra flavor.

N.V.: Calories: 250 per serving, Fat: 10g, Carbs: 10g, Protein: 30g, Sugar: 2g

GRILLED LEMON BASIL CHICKEN SKEWERS

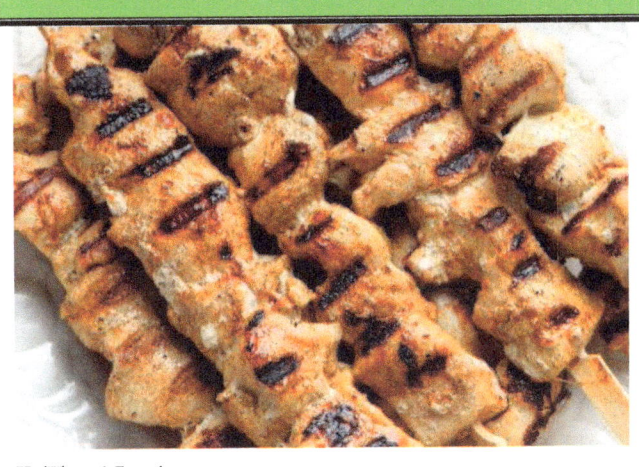

P.T.: 15 min
C.T.: 10 min
M.C: Grilling
SERVINGS: 4
INGR:

- 1.5 lbs boneless, skinless chicken breasts, cubed
- 1/4 Cup olive oil
- 2 Tbsp lemon juice
- 2 cloves garlic, minced
- 1/4 Cup fresh basil, chopped
- Salt and pepper to taste
- Wooden skewers, soaked in water

DIRECTIONS:

1. In a bowl, whisk together olive oil, lemon juice, garlic, basil, salt, and pepper.
2. Add chicken cubes and marinate for at least 30 minutes.
3. Thread chicken onto skewers.
4. Preheat grill to medium-high heat.
5. Grill skewers for 5-7 minutes on each side or until cooked through.
6. Serve immediately, garnished with additional basil.

TIPS:

- Serve with a side of tzatziki sauce.
- Add vegetables like bell peppers or onions to the skewers.

N.V.: Calories: 320 per serving, Fat: 16g, Carbs: 2g, Protein: 40g, Sugar: 0g

LEMON HERB TILAPIA

P.T.: 10 min
C.T.: 15 min
M.C: Baking
SERVINGS: 4
INGR:

- 4 tilapia fillets
- 2 Tbsp olive oil
- 1 lemon, juiced and zested
- 2 cloves garlic, minced
- 1 Tsp dried parsley
- 1 Tsp dried thyme
- Salt and pepper to taste

DIRECTIONS:

1. Preheat oven to 375°F (190°C).
2. In a bowl, mix olive oil, lemon juice, lemon zest, garlic, parsley, thyme, salt, and pepper.
3. Place tilapia fillets on a baking sheet and brush with lemon herb mixture.
4. Bake for 12-15 minutes or until fish flakes easily with a fork.
5. Serve hot, garnished with lemon slices.

TIPS:

- Serve with steamed vegetables or quinoa.
- Substitute tilapia with cod or haddock.

N.V.: Calories: 280 per serving, Fat: 14g, Carbs: 2g, Protein: 36g, Sugar: 0g

2. VEGETABLE-CENTRIC MEALS

STUFFED BELL PEPPERS WITH QUINOA AND BLACK BEANS

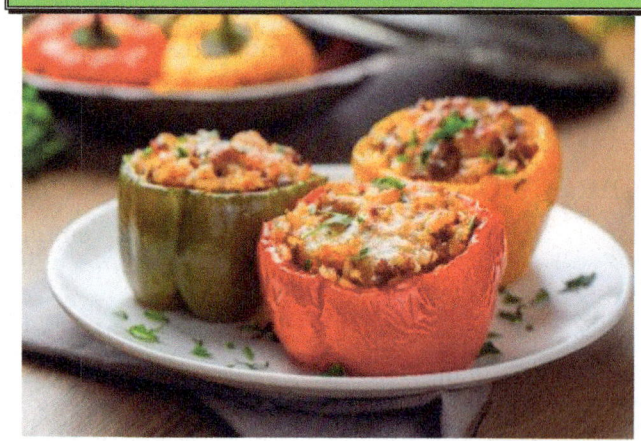

P.T.: 15 min
C.T.: 30 min
M.C: Baking
SERVINGS: 4
INGR:

- 4 large bell peppers, halved and seeded
- 1 Cup quinoa, rinsed
- 2 Cups vegetable broth
- 1 can (15 oz) black beans, drained and rinsed
- 1 Cup corn kernels
- 1 Cup diced tomatoes
- 1 Tsp cumin
- 1 Tsp chili powder
- 1/4 Cup fresh cilantro, chopped
- Salt and pepper to taste
- 1/2 Cup shredded cheddar cheese

DIRECTIONS:

1. Preheat oven to 375°F (190°C).
2. In a saucepan, bring quinoa and vegetable broth to a boil. Reduce heat, cover, and simmer for 15 minutes.
3. In a large bowl, combine cooked quinoa, black beans, corn, tomatoes, cumin, chili powder, cilantro, salt, and pepper.
4. Fill each bell pepper half with the quinoa mixture and place in a baking dish.
5. Sprinkle with cheddar cheese.
6. Bake for 25-30 minutes or until peppers are tender.

TIPS:

- Use different colored bell peppers for a

vibrant dish.
- Add avocado slices for extra creaminess.

N.V.: Calories: 350 per serving, Fat: 10g, Carbs: 55g, Protein: 15g, Sugar: 8g

RATATOUILLE

P.T.: 20 min
C.T.: 45 min
M.C: Stovetop
SERVINGS: 6
INGR:
- 1 eggplant, diced
- 2 zucchini, sliced
- 1 red bell pepper, diced
- 1 yellow bell pepper, diced
- 1 onion, chopped
- 4 cloves garlic, minced
- 2 Cup s tomatoes, diced
- 2 Tbsp olive oil
- 1 Tsp dried thyme
- 1 Tsp dried oregano
- Salt and pepper to taste
- 1/4 Cup fresh basil, chopped

DIRECTIONS:
1. Heat olive oil in a large pot over medium heat. Add onion and garlic, sauté until translucent.
2. Add eggplant, zucchini, bell peppers, thyme, oregano, salt, and pepper. Cook for 10 minutes.
3. Stir in tomatoes and bring to a simmer. Cover and cook for 30 minutes or until vegetables are tender.
4. Stir in fresh basil before serving.

TIPS:
- Serve over pasta or rice for a heartier meal.
- Top with Parmesan cheese for added flavor.

N.V.: Calories: 180 per serving, Fat: 7g, Carbs: 28g, Protein: 4g, Sugar: 12g

SPAGHETTI SQUASH WITH MARINARA SAUCE

P.T.: 10 min
C.T.: 40 min
M.C: Baking/Stovetop
SERVINGS: 4
INGR:
- 1 large spaghetti squash
- 2 Cup s marinara sauce
- 1/4 Cup Parmesan cheese, grated
- 1 Tbsp olive oil
- Salt and pepper to taste
- Fresh basil for garnish

DIRECTIONS:
1. Preheat oven to 400°F (204°C).
2. Cut spaghetti squash in half lengthwise and scoop out seeds.
3. Drizzle olive oil on the squash halves and season with salt and pepper.
4. Place cut side down on a baking sheet and bake for 30-40 minutes until tender.
5. Use a fork to scrape out the spaghetti strands.
6. Heat marinara sauce in a saucepan. Serve over spaghetti squash and top with Parmesan cheese and basil.

TIPS:
- Add sautéed mushrooms for extra flavor.
- Substitute marinara with pesto for a different taste.

N.V.: Calories: 220 per serving, Fat: 10g, Carbs: 30g, Protein: 6g, Sugar: 12g

CAULIFLOWER FRIED RICE

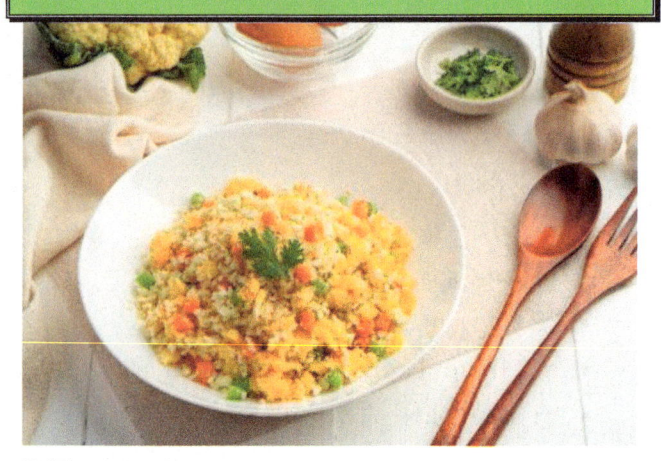

P.T.: 10 min
C.T.: 15 min
M.C: Stovetop
SERVINGS: 4
INGR:

- 1 head cauliflower, grated into rice-size pieces
- 1 Cup peas and carrots, frozen
- 1/2 Cup onion, chopped
- 2 cloves garlic, minced
- 2 Tbsp soy sauce
- 2 eggs, beaten
- 2 Tbsp sesame oil
- 1/4 Cup green onions, sliced
- Salt and pepper to taste

DIRECTIONS:

1. Heat sesame oil in a large skillet over medium heat. Add onion and garlic, sauté until fragrant.
2. Add peas and carrots, cook for 3 minutes.
3. Stir in cauliflower rice and soy sauce, cook for 5 minutes or until cauliflower is tender.
4. Push cauliflower to one side, pour beaten eggs on the other side. Scramble and mix into cauliflower.
5. Season with salt and pepper, garnish with green onions.

TIPS:

- Add cooked chicken or shrimp for more protein.
- Use coconut aminos for a soy-free option.

N.V.: Calories: 150 per serving, Fat: 8g, Carbs: 14g, Protein: 6g, Sugar: 5g

ZUCCHINI NOODLES WITH PESTO

P.T.: 10 min
C.T.: 5 min
M.C: Stovetop
SERVINGS: 4
INGR:

- 4 large zucchinis, spiralized
- 1/2 Cup pesto sauce
- 1/4 Cup cherry tomatoes, halved
- 1/4 Cup Parmesan cheese, grated
- 1 Tbsp olive oil
- Salt and pepper to taste

DIRECTIONS:

1. Heat olive oil in a large skillet over medium heat.
2. Add zucchini noodles and cook for 2-3 minutes until just tender.
3. Stir in pesto sauce and cherry tomatoes.
4. Season with salt and pepper, top with Parmesan cheese.

TIPS:

- Add grilled chicken for extra protein.
- Substitute zucchini with spiralized carrots or beets.

N.V.: Calories: 250 per serving, Fat: 20g, Carbs: 14g, Protein: 6g, Sugar: 4g

EGGPLANT PARMESAN

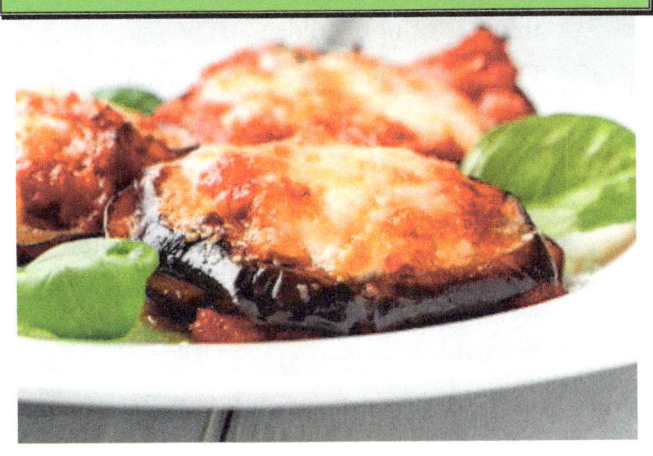

P.T.: 15 min
C.T.: 45 min
M.C: Baking
SERVINGS: 6
INGR:

- 2 large eggplants, sliced
- 2 Cup s marinara sauce
- 1 Cup mozzarella cheese, shredded
- 1/2 Cup Parmesan cheese, grated
- 1 Cup bread crumbs
- 2 eggs, beaten
- 1/4 Cup olive oil
- Salt and pepper to taste

DIRECTIONS:

1. Preheat oven to 375°F (190°C).
2. Dip eggplant slices in beaten eggs, then coat with bread crumbs.
3. Heat olive oil in a skillet over medium heat. Fry eggplant until golden on both sides.
4. In a baking dish, layer marinara sauce, fried eggplant, mozzarella, and Parmesan cheese.
5. Repeat layers and finish with cheese on top.
6. Bake for 30 minutes or until cheese is bubbly and golden.

TIPS:

- Use gluten-free bread crumbs if needed.
- Serve with a side salad for a complete meal.

N.V.: Calories: 400 per serving, Fat: 22g, Carbs: 38g, Protein: 15g, Sugar: 9g

VEGGIE STIR-FRY WITH TOFU

P.T.: 10 min
C.T.: 15 min
M.C: Stovetop
SERVINGS: 4
INGR:

- 1 block (14 oz) firm tofu, cubed
- 1 red bell pepper, sliced
- 1 Cup broccoli florets
- 1 Cup snap peas
- 1 carrot, julienned
- 2 Tbsp soy sauce
- 1 Tbsp sesame oil
- 1 clove garlic, minced
- 1 Tsp ginger, grated
- Salt and pepper to taste
- Sesame seeds for garnish

DIRECTIONS:

1. Heat sesame oil in a large skillet over medium heat.
2. Add garlic and ginger, sauté until fragrant.
3. Add tofu and cook until golden brown.
4. Stir in bell pepper, broccoli, snap peas, and carrot. Cook for 5 minutes.
5. Add soy sauce, toss to coat vegetables.
6. Season with salt and pepper, garnish with sesame seeds.

TIPS:

- Serve over brown rice or quinoa.
- Add your favorite vegetables for variety.

N.V.: Calories: 280 per serving, Fat: 16g, Carbs: 20g, Protein: 16g, Sugar: 4g

3. COMFORT FOODS MADE HEALTHY

CAULIFLOWER MAC AND CHEESE

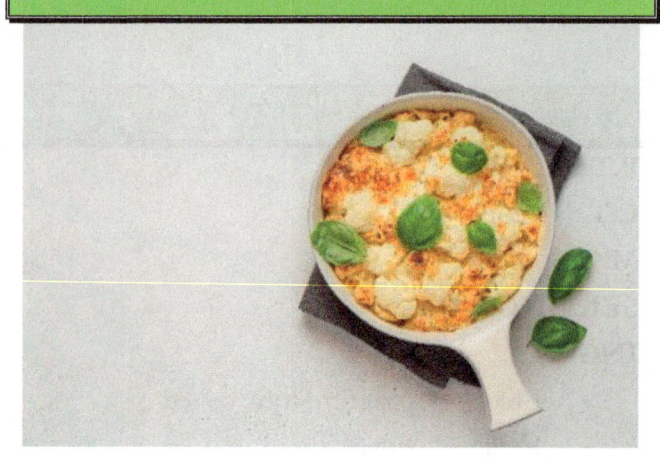

P.T.: 10 min
C.T.: 30 min
M.C: Baking
SERVINGS: 4
INGR:

- 1 head cauliflower, cut into florets
- 2 Cup s shredded cheddar cheese
- 1 Cup milk
- 2 Tbsp butter
- 2 Tbsp all-purpose flour
- 1/2 Tsp garlic powder
- Salt and pepper to taste
- 1/4 Cup breadcrumbs
- 2 Tbsp chopped parsley for garnish

DIRECTIONS:

1. Preheat oven to 375°F (190°C).
2. Steam cauliflower florets until tender, about 10 minutes.
3. In a saucepan, melt butter over medium heat. Whisk in flour to form a roux and cook for 1 minute.
4. Gradually whisk in milk, cooking until thickened. Stir in cheddar cheese, garlic powder, salt, and pepper until cheese is melted.
5. Mix cheese sauce with cauliflower and transfer to a baking dish.
6. Top with breadcrumbs and bake for 15 minutes or until golden.
7. Garnish with chopped parsley before serving.

TIPS:

- Add a pinch of cayenne pepper for a spicy kick.
- Use gluten-free flour and breadcrumbs if needed.

N.V.: Calories: 320 per serving, Fat: 22g, Carbs: 16g, Protein: 18g, Sugar: 5g

TURKEY AND SWEET POTATO SHEPHERD'S PIE

P.T.: 15 min
C.T.: 30 min
M.C: Baking
SERVINGS: 4
INGR:

- 1 lb ground turkey
- 2 large sweet potatoes, peeled and cubed
- 1 onion, diced
- 2 cloves garlic, minced
- 1 Cup peas and carrots, frozen
- 1 Cup chicken broth
- 2 Tbsp olive oil
- 1 Tbsp tomato paste
- 1 Tsp dried thyme
- Salt and pepper to taste

DIRECTIONS:

1. Preheat oven to 400°F (204°C).
2. Boil sweet potatoes until tender, then mash with 1 Tbsp olive oil, salt, and pepper.
3. In a skillet, heat remaining olive oil and sauté onion and garlic until soft.
4. Add ground turkey, cook until browned. Stir in tomato paste, chicken broth, thyme, salt, and pepper.
5. Add peas and carrots, cook for 5 minutes. Transfer to a baking dish.

6. Spread mashed sweet potatoes over the turkey mixture.
7. Bake for 15 minutes or until top is golden.

TIPS:
- Substitute sweet potatoes with regular potatoes for a classic version.
- Add a sprinkle of cheese on top for extra flavor.

N.V.: Calories: 360 per serving, Fat: 14g, Carbs: 40g, Protein: 26g, Sugar: 8g

QUINOA AND VEGETABLE STUFFED PEPPERS

P.T.: 15 min
C.T.: 30 min
M.C: Baking
SERVINGS: 4
INGR:

- 4 large bell peppers, halved and seeded
- 1 Cup quinoa, rinsed
- 2 Cup s vegetable broth
- 1 zucchini, diced
- 1 Cup mushrooms, diced
- 1 onion, chopped
- 2 cloves garlic, minced
- 1 can (15 oz) diced tomatoes, drained
- 1 Tsp dried oregano
- Salt and pepper to taste
- 1/4 Cup grated Parmesan cheese

DIRECTIONS:
1. Preheat oven to 375°F (190°C).
2. Cook quinoa in vegetable broth according to package instructions.
3. In a skillet, sauté onion, garlic, zucchini, and mushrooms until soft.
4. Stir in cooked quinoa, diced tomatoes, oregano, salt, and pepper.
5. Fill each pepper half with quinoa mixture and place in a baking dish.
6. Sprinkle with Parmesan cheese and bake for 25-30 minutes.

TIPS:
- Use different colored peppers for variety.
- Add fresh basil for extra flavor.

N.V.: Calories: 340 per serving, Fat: 10g, Carbs: 50g, Protein: 12g, Sugar: 8g

HEALTHY CHICKEN PARMESAN

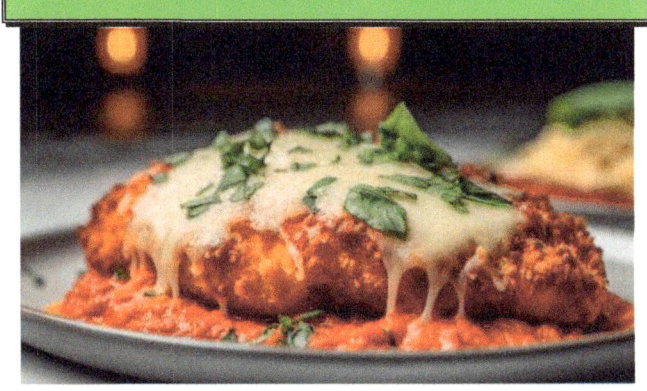

P.T.: 15 min
C.T.: 25 min
M.C: Baking
SERVINGS: 4
INGR:

- 4 boneless, skinless chicken breasts
- 1 Cup marinara sauce
- 1 Cup mozzarella cheese, shredded
- 1/2 Cup Parmesan cheese, grated
- 1 Cup whole wheat breadcrumbs
- 2 eggs, beaten
- 2 Tbsp olive oil
- Salt and pepper to taste
- Fresh basil for garnish

DIRECTIONS:
1. Preheat oven to 400°F (204°C).
2. Dip chicken breasts in beaten eggs, then coat with breadcrumbs.
3. Heat olive oil in a skillet over medium heat and brown chicken on both sides.
4. Place chicken in a baking dish, top with marinara sauce, mozzarella, and Parmesan cheese.
5. Bake for 15-20 minutes or until cheese is melted and bubbly.

6. Garnish with fresh basil before serving.

TIPS:
- Serve with whole wheat pasta for a complete meal.
- Use gluten-free breadcrumbs if needed.

N.V.: Calories: 380 per serving, Fat: 20g, Carbs: 20g, Protein: 32g, Sugar: 5g

Veggie Lasagna with Zucchini Noodles

P.T.: 20 min
C.T.: 40 min
M.C: Baking
SERVINGS: 6
INGR:
- 3 large zucchinis, sliced lengthwise
- 1 Cup ricotta cheese
- 1 egg
- 2 Cup s marinara sauce
- 1 Cup mozzarella cheese, shredded
- 1/2 Cup Parmesan cheese, grated
- 1 Cup spinach, chopped
- 1/4 Cup fresh basil, chopped
- Salt and pepper to taste

DIRECTIONS:
1. Preheat oven to 375°F (190°C).
2. Mix ricotta cheese, egg, spinach, basil, salt, and pepper in a bowl.
3. Spread a thin layer of marinara sauce in a baking dish.
4. Layer zucchini slices, ricotta mixture, marinara sauce, and mozzarella cheese. Repeat layers.
5. Top with Parmesan cheese and bake for 30-40 minutes or until bubbly.
6. Let cool for 5 minutes before serving.

TIPS:
- Use a mandoline for evenly sliced zucchini.
- Add mushrooms or eggplant for more vegetables.

N.V.: Calories: 310 per serving, Fat: 18g, Carbs: 18g, Protein: 22g, Sugar: 8g

Baked Sweet Potato Fries with Avocado Dip

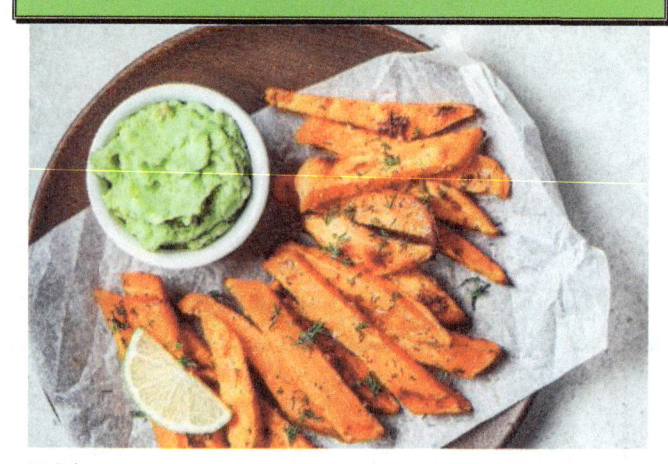

P.T.: 10 min
C.T.: 30 min
M.C: Baking
SERVINGS: 4
INGR:
- 3 large sweet potatoes, cut into fries
- 2 Tbsp olive oil
- 1 Tsp paprika
- Salt and pepper to taste
- 2 avocados, peeled and pitted
- 1 lime, juiced
- 1/4 Cup Greek yogurt
- 1 clove garlic, minced

DIRECTIONS:
1. Preheat oven to 425°F (220°C).
2. Toss sweet potatoes with olive oil, paprika, salt, and pepper. Spread on a baking sheet.
3. Bake for 25-30 minutes, turning halfway, until crispy.
4. In a blender, combine avocados, lime juice, Greek yogurt, garlic, salt, and pepper. Blend until smooth.
5. Serve sweet potato fries with avocado dip.

TIPS:
- Add a pinch of cayenne pepper to fries for

heat.
- Use sour cream instead of Greek yogurt if preferred.

N.V.: Calories: 340 per serving, Fat: 22g, Carbs: 35g, Protein: 4g, Sugar: 8g

LENTIL AND VEGETABLE SHEPHERD'S PIE

P.T.: 15 min
C.T.: 45 min
M.C: Baking
SERVINGS: 6
INGR:
- 1 Cup lentils, rinsed
- 2 Cups vegetable broth
- 2 carrots, diced
- 1 onion, diced
- 2 cloves garlic, minced
- 1 Cup peas
- 1 Tbsp olive oil
- 1 Tbsp tomato paste
- 1 Tsp thyme
- Salt and pepper to taste
- 4 potatoes, peeled and cubed
- 1/4 Cup milk
- 2 Tbsp butter

DIRECTIONS:
1. Preheat oven to 375°F (190°C).
2. Cook lentils in vegetable broth until tender, about 20 minutes.
3. In a skillet, heat olive oil and sauté onion, garlic, and carrots until soft. Stir in tomato paste, thyme, salt, and pepper.
4. Add cooked lentils and peas. Transfer to a baking dish.
5. Boil potatoes until tender, then mash with milk, butter, salt, and pepper.
6. Spread mashed potatoes over the lentil mixture.
7. Bake for 25 minutes or until golden.

TIPS:
- Use sweet potatoes for a sweeter topping.
- Add mushrooms for more depth of flavor.

N.V.: Calories: 380 per serving, Fat: 10g, Carbs: 65g, Protein: 12g, Sugar: 6g

CHAPTER 7: DESSERTS AND TREATS
1. LOW-CALORIE DESSERTS

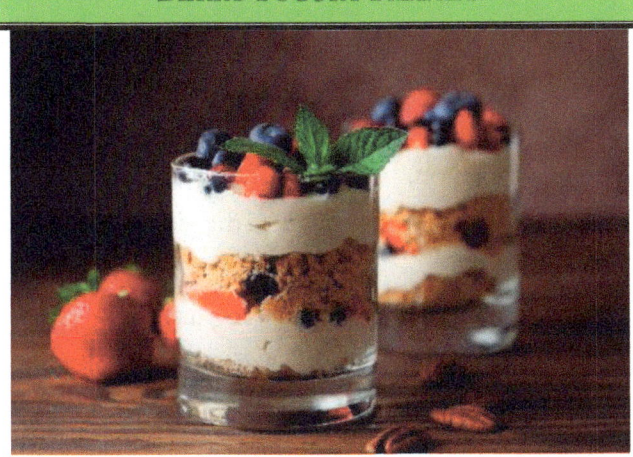

BERRY YOGURT PARFAIT

P.T.: 10 min
C.T.: 0 min
M.C: None
SERVINGS: 4
INGR:
- 2 Cup s Greek yogurt, non-fat
- 1 Cup mixed berries (strawberries, blueberries, raspberries)
- 1/2 Cup granola
- 2 Tbsp honey
- 1 Tsp vanilla extract

DIRECTIONS:
1. In a bowl, mix Greek yogurt with honey and vanilla extract.
2. In serving glasses, layer 1/4 Cup yogurt mixture, followed by a layer of berries and a layer of granola.
3. Repeat the layers until all ingredients are used.
4. Top with a few berries and a drizzle of honey.

TIPS:
- Use seasonal berries for the freshest flavor.
- Substitute granola with crushed nuts for a lower-carb option.

N.V.: Calories: 160 per serving, Fat: 2g, Carbs: 27g, Protein: 10g, Sugar: 16g

CHOCOLATE AVOCADO MOUSSE

P.T.: 10 min
C.T.: 0 min
M.C: None
SERVINGS: 4
INGR:
- 2 ripe avocados, peeled and pitted
- 1/4 Cup cocoa powder, unsweetened
- 1/4 Cup honey
- 1/4 Cup almond milk, unsweetened
- 1 Tsp vanilla extract
- Pinch of salt

DIRECTIONS:
1. In a blender, combine avocados, cocoa powder, honey, almond milk, vanilla extract, and salt.
2. Blend until smooth and creamy.
3. Spoon mousse into serving bowls.
4. Refrigerate for at least 30 minutes before serving.

TIPS:
- Garnish with fresh berries or mint leaves for added freshness.
- Adjust sweetness by adding more honey if desired.

N.V.: Calories: 180 per serving, Fat: 11g, Carbs: 24g, Protein: 3g, Sugar: 16g

BAKED APPLES WITH CINNAMON

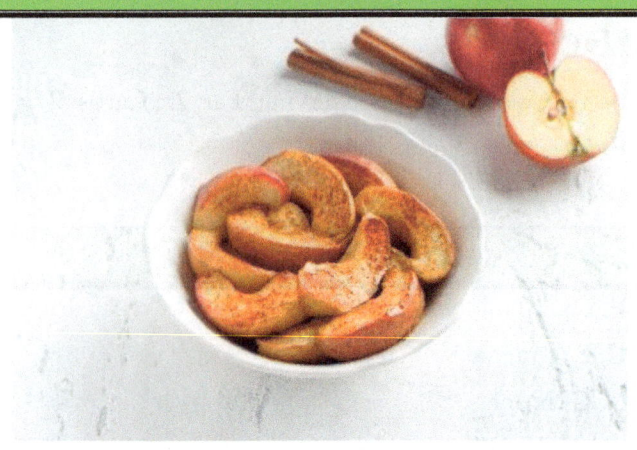

P.T.: 10 min
C.T.: 25 min
M.C: Baking
SERVINGS: 4
INGR:

- 4 medium apples, cored
- 1/4 Cup raisins
- 1/4 Cup chopped walnuts
- 2 Tbsp honey
- 1 Tsp ground cinnamon
- 1/2 Cup water

DIRECTIONS:

1. Preheat oven to 350°F (175°C).
2. Place cored apples in a baking dish.
3. In a bowl, mix raisins, walnuts, honey, and cinnamon.
4. Stuff the mixture into the center of each apple.
5. Pour water into the baking dish.
6. Bake for 25 minutes or until apples are tender.

TIPS:

- Serve warm with a dollop of Greek yogurt.
- Use different nuts, like pecans or almonds, for variety.

N.V.: Calories: 150 per serving, Fat: 5g, Carbs: 28g, Protein: 1g, Sugar: 20g

2. HEALTHY BAKING

ALMOND FLOUR BANANA BREAD

P.T.: 10 min
C.T.: 45 min
M.C: Baking
SERVINGS: 8
INGR:

- 2 Cup s almond flour
- 3 ripe bananas, mashed
- 3 large eggs
- 1/4 Cup honey
- 1 Tsp vanilla extract
- 1 Tsp baking soda
- 1/2 Tsp cinnamon
- 1/4 Tsp salt
- 1/4 Cup walnuts, chopped (optional)

DIRECTIONS:

1. Preheat oven to 350°F (175°C). Grease a loaf pan or line it with parchment paper.
2. In a large bowl, mix mashed bananas, eggs, honey, and vanilla extract until smooth.
3. In another bowl, combine almond flour, baking soda, cinnamon, and salt.
4. Gradually add the dry ingredients to the wet ingredients, stirring until well combined.
5. Fold in walnuts if using.
6. Pour the batter into the prepared loaf pan.
7. Bake for 45 minutes or until a toothpick inserted into the center comes out clean.
8. Let cool before slicing and serving.

TIPS:

- Add chocolate chips for extra sweetness.
- Use pecans instead of walnuts for a different flavor.

N.V.: Calories: 210 per serving, Fat: 14g, Carbs: 17g, Protein: 6g, Sugar: 10g

Whole Wheat Blueberry Muffins

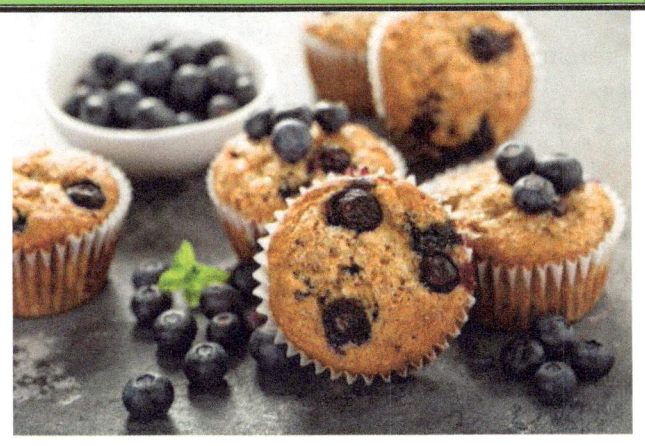

P.T.: 10 min
C.T.: 20 min
M.C: Baking
SERVINGS: 12
INGR:
- 1 1/2 Cup s whole wheat flour
- 1/2 Cup rolled oats
- 1/2 Cup honey
- 1/3 Cup coconut oil, melted
- 1/2 Cup almond milk
- 1 Tsp vanilla extract
- 1 Tsp baking powder
- 1/2 Tsp baking soda
- 1/2 Tsp cinnamon
- 1/4 Tsp salt
- 1 Cup blueberries

DIRECTIONS:
1. Preheat oven to 375°F (190°C). Line a muffin tin with paper liners.
2. In a large bowl, whisk together flour, oats, baking powder, baking soda, cinnamon, and salt.
3. In another bowl, mix honey, coconut oil, almond milk, and vanilla extract.
4. Pour wet ingredients into dry ingredients and stir until just combined.
5. Gently fold in blueberries.
6. Divide batter evenly among muffin Cup s.
7. Bake for 18-20 minutes or until a toothpick inserted in the center comes out clean.
8. Let cool in the pan for 5 minutes, then transfer to a wire rack to cool completely.

TIPS:
- Use fresh or frozen blueberries.
- Add a sprinkle of oats on top before baking for added texture.

N.V.: Calories: 150 per serving, Fat: 6g, Carbs: 23g, Protein: 3g, Sugar: 10g

Chocolate Chip Oatmeal Cookies

P.T.: 10 min
C.T.: 12 min
M.C: Baking
SERVINGS: 24 cookies
INGR:
- 1 Cup rolled oats
- 1 Cup whole wheat flour
- 1/2 Cup coconut oil, melted
- 1/2 Cup honey
- 1 large egg
- 1 Tsp vanilla extract
- 1/2 Tsp baking soda
- 1/4 Tsp salt
- 1/2 Cup dark chocolate chips

DIRECTIONS:
1. Preheat oven to 350°F (175°C). Line a baking sheet with parchment paper.
2. In a large bowl, combine oats, flour, baking soda, and salt.
3. In another bowl, whisk together coconut oil, honey, egg, and vanilla extract.
4. Pour wet ingredients into dry ingredients and stir until well combined.
5. Fold in chocolate chips.
6. Drop tablespoon-sized scoops of dough onto the prepared baking sheet.
7. Bake for 10-12 minutes or until edges are golden brown.
8. Let cool on the baking sheet for 5 minutes

before transferring to a wire rack to cool completely.

TIPS:
- Use raisins or dried cranberries instead of chocolate chips for a different flavor.
- Add a pinch of cinnamon for extra warmth.

N.V.: Calories: 120 per cookie, Fat: 7g, Carbs: 15g, Protein: 2g, Sugar: 8g

3. INDULGENT YET GUILT-FREE

CHOCOLATE PEANUT BUTTER CUPS

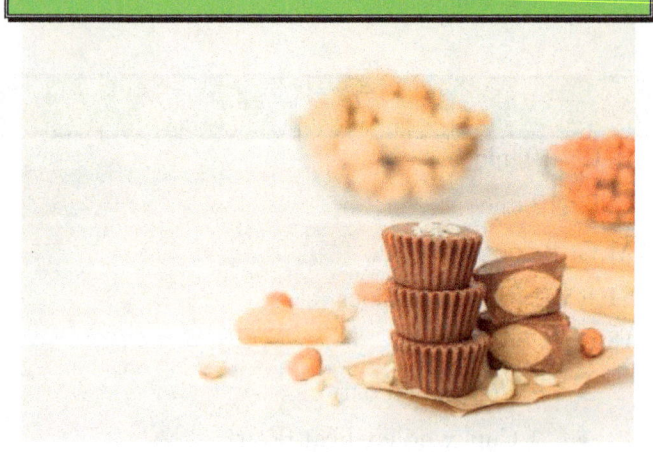

P.T.: 10 min
C.T.: 0 min (Chill for 30 min)
M.C: None
SERVINGS: 12 Cups
INGR:
- 1/2 Cup natural peanut butter
- 1/4 Cup coconut oil, melted
- 1/4 Cup honey
- 1 Tsp vanilla extract
- 1/4 Tsp salt
- 1/2 Cup dark chocolate chips

DIRECTIONS:
1. In a bowl, mix peanut butter, coconut oil, honey, vanilla extract, and salt until smooth.
2. Melt chocolate chips in a microwave-safe bowl in 30-second intervals until smooth.
3. Line a muffin tin with paper liners. Spoon 1 Tsp of melted chocolate into the bottom of each liner.
4. Top with a spoonful of the peanut butter mixture, then add another Tsp of chocolate on top.
5. Chill in the refrigerator for at least 30 minutes or until set.

TIPS:
- Use almond butter for a different flavor.
- Sprinkle a pinch of sea salt on top for added taste.

N.V.: Calories: 120 per Cup, Fat: 9g, Carbs: 8g, Protein: 3g, Sugar: 6g

CHAPTER 8: STAYING MOTIVATED
1. Maintaining Momentum

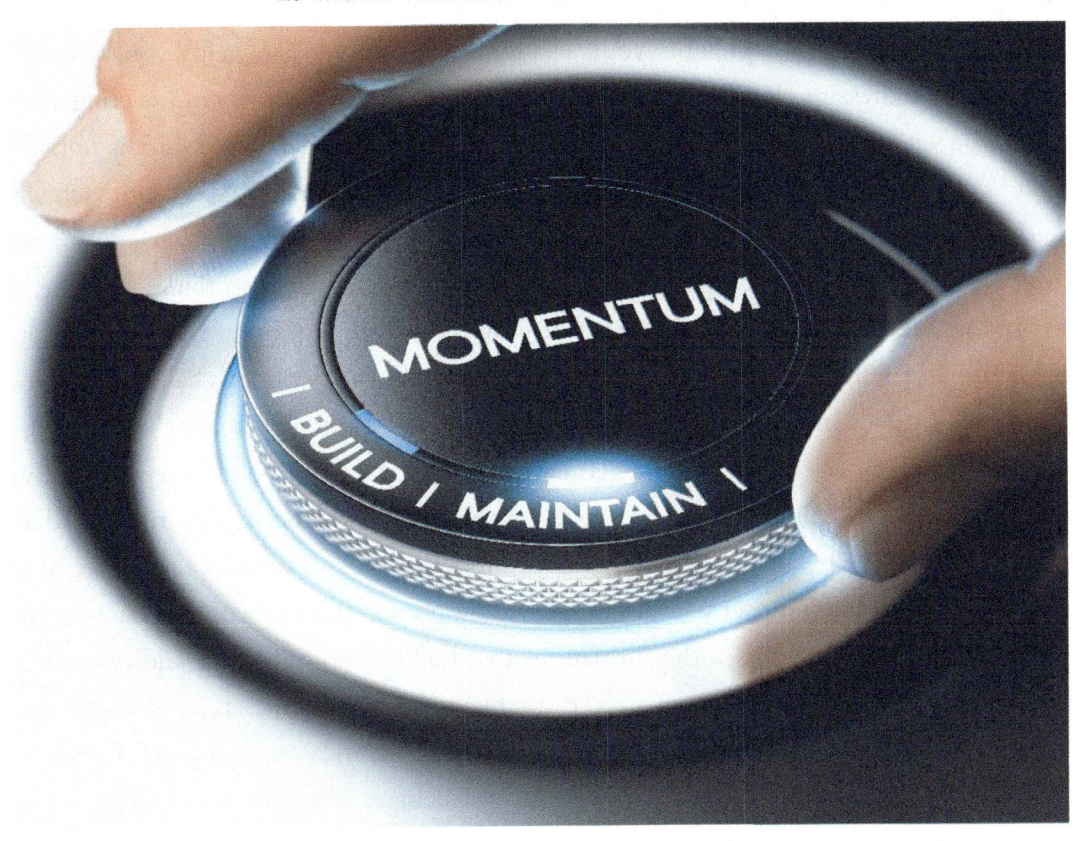

Maintaining momentum in a weight loss journey is much like keeping a well-tended garden; it requires consistency, attention, and a bit of creativity. Every day is an opportunity to nurture your progress, and the process can be just as rewarding as the results. As you embark on this path, consider the ways you can build a lifestyle that not only embraces healthy habits but also fosters a mindset that keeps you moving forward, even when challenges arise. Picture your journey as a marathon, not a sprint. It's a steady-paced adventure where endurance counts more than speed. This mindset helps in understanding that temporary setbacks are just that—temporary. They do not define your entire journey or your capability to succeed. Embracing this perspective makes it easier to keep pushing forward, to continue placing one foot in front of the other even when the path seems uphill. One of the most effective ways to maintain momentum is by setting clear, achievable goals. Imagine these goals as signposts along your journey. They guide you, providing motivation and a sense of direction. Whether it's losing a certain number of pounds or fitting into a favorite outfit, these benchmarks offer tangible reminders of what you're working towards. However, it's crucial that these goals are realistic and aligned with your lifestyle. This doesn't mean they shouldn't be ambitious; they should be just challenging enough to keep you motivated but not so daunting that they seem unattainable. Visualize your success. Imagine reaching your goals and how it will make you feel. What will your day-to-day life look like? What activities will you enjoy that you might not be able to do now? This visualization can be a powerful motivator. It acts as a mental rehearsal for success, keeping your desired outcomes at the forefront of your mind. Your support system plays a vital role in maintaining momentum. Whether it's friends, family, or a community group, having people who understand your journey and can offer encouragement is invaluable. They are your cheerleaders, celebrating your successes and lifting you up during difficult times. Don't hesitate to reach out and share your journey with them. You might find that their stories and experiences offer insights that could help you, too. Another key aspect of maintaining momentum is to track your progress. This doesn't just mean stepping on the scale. Consider keeping a journal where you record your achievements, how you're feeling, and any obstacles you encounter. This practice not only highlights your accomplishments but also helps you identify patterns or triggers that may need addressing. Reflecting on your progress can be incredibly empowering and can remind you just how far you've come. It's also important to remain flexible and adaptable. Life is unpredictable, and there will be times when things don't go as planned. Learning to adapt and adjust your approach without giving up is a hallmark of maintaining momentum. This flexibility allows you to continue your journey without being derailed by unforeseen challenges. Incorporate variety into your routine to keep things exciting. Whether it's trying a new workout, experimenting with different healthy recipes, or exploring new hobbies that keep you active, variety helps prevent monotony. It keeps your mind engaged and your body challenged. Remember, your journey should be enjoyable and fulfilling. Celebrating your achievements, no matter how small, is essential. Each milestone reached is a testament to your hard work and dedication. Take time to acknowledge these victories, whether it's treating yourself to a non-food reward like a new book or a relaxing day out. These celebrations reinforce positive behaviors and motivate you to keep going. Consider the power of affirmations. Positive self-talk can significantly impact your motivation and outlook. Remind yourself daily of your strengths and abilities. Replace negative thoughts with affirmations that build your confidence and resolve. This practice shifts your focus from what you can't do to what you can achieve. Finding balance is another critical component. It's easy to become consumed by the numbers on the scale or the calories on your plate. Remember to take a step back and view the bigger picture. Your health and well-being encompass more than just weight. They include your mental and emotional state, your energy levels, and your overall happiness. Strive for a balanced approach that nourishes both body and soul. Finally, remember that setbacks are part of the journey. They are not a reflection of your worth or your ability to succeed. Instead of seeing them as failures, view them as opportunities to learn and grow. Analyze what went wrong, adjust your plan, and continue forward with renewed determination. Each setback is a stepping stone, guiding you closer to your goals.

2. Overcoming Challenges

Imagine your journey as climbing a mountain. The peak represents your ultimate goal, whether it's a target weight, a specific health milestone, or simply a healthier lifestyle. The path is steep and daunting at times, but the view from the top is worth every step. Challenges along the way are like rocky outcrops or sudden storms. They may slow your progress, but they also provide opportunities to grow stronger and more determined. One of the first hurdles many face is the temptation to revert to old habits, especially when progress seems slow. It's important to remember that change takes time and patience. Old habits didn't form overnight, and new ones won't either. When you find yourself tempted, take a moment to reflect on why you started this journey. Reconnect with your reasons and visualize the benefits you will enjoy once you reach your goals. This mental exercise can be a powerful motivator, helping you push past momentary cravings or laziness. Stress is another common challenge. Life is full of unexpected events that can throw off your routine. Stress can trigger emotional eating or a lapse in your healthy habits. It's crucial to develop strategies for managing stress that don't involve food. Consider incorporating activities like yoga, meditation, or even a brisk walk to clear your mind. These practices not only help manage stress but also boost your overall well-being.

A lack of support can also feel like a stumbling block. While many are fortunate to have family and friends who cheer them on, others may not find the same level of encouragement. If this is your situation, seek out communities that share your goals. Online forums, local support groups, or fitness classes can provide the camaraderie and motivation you need. Connecting with others who understand your struggles can be incredibly empowering, offering a sense of belonging and encouragement. Plateaus are perhaps one of the most frustrating challenges. You're doing everything right—eating well, exercising regularly—but the scale stubbornly refuses to budge. Remember, plateaus are a natural part of the weight loss process. They happen to everyone and are often a sign that your body is adjusting to a new normal. Instead of getting discouraged, use this time to evaluate your habits. Are you truly sticking to your plan? Is your body accustomed to your exercise routine? Perhaps it's time to shake things up. Try a new workout, adjust your calorie intake slightly, or focus on different types of exercises to surprise your body and reignite your progress. Another challenge is the perception of failure. We all have setbacks, whether it's an unplanned indulgence or a missed workout. The key is not to view these as failures but as learning experiences. Reflect on what led to the setback and how you can prevent it in the future. Maybe you need to find healthier alternatives for your favorite treats or adjust your schedule to ensure time for exercise. Every setback is an opportunity to refine your approach and strengthen your resolve. Time constraints are a reality for many people, making it difficult to prioritize health and wellness. In our fast-paced world, it can feel like there aren't enough hours in the day to cook healthy meals or fit in a workout. The solution lies in effective time management and finding efficiencies that work for you. Meal prepping is a great way to ensure you always have healthy options available, even on your busiest days. Planning your workouts as you would any important appointment can also help keep your fitness routine on track. Boredom can also derail progress. Eating the same meals or following the same workout routine can become monotonous, sapping motivation. To keep things exciting, challenge yourself to try new recipes or explore different cuisines that fit your dietary needs. Vary your workouts by trying a new sport, joining a class, or exploring nature trails for a change of scenery. Keeping things fresh and exciting helps maintain your enthusiasm and commitment. Sometimes, the challenge is deeper, rooted in self-doubt or negative self-talk. It's essential to address these internal obstacles, as they can undermine your efforts from within. Practice self-compassion and recognize that you are worthy of success and happiness. Replace negative thoughts with affirmations that reinforce your strength and determination. Over time, this positive mindset will become a powerful ally in overcoming challenges. Finally, remember to celebrate your progress, no matter how small it may seem. Every pound lost, every healthier choice, every mile walked is a step closer to your goal. Acknowledge these victories and reward yourself in ways that support your journey, whether it's a relaxing bath, a new book, or a day spent doing something you love. Overcoming challenges is an integral part of your weight loss journey, shaping you into a stronger, more resilient version of yourself. Embrace the process, knowing that every obstacle overcome is a testament to your determination and commitment. With the right mindset and strategies, you can conquer any challenge and continue forward, closer each day to the healthier life you envision. Your journey is a testament to your strength and dedication, and each challenge is simply another opportunity to prove to yourself just how capable you truly are.

3. Long-Term Success

Reaching your weight loss goals is a momentous achievement, one that deserves celebration and recognition. But the journey doesn't end there. In many ways, the true challenge begins with maintaining those hard-earned results for the long term. This stage requires a shift in focus, from the effort of losing weight to the art of sustaining a healthy lifestyle that supports your physical and mental well-being. Imagine your journey like tending to a flourishing garden. The initial work of planting and nurturing has paid off, and now it's time to ensure your garden thrives for years to come. This involves continuous care and attention, adapting to changes in weather, and preventing new weeds from taking root. Similarly, achieving long-term success in weight management is about cultivating habits that become second nature and making adjustments as life evolves. The first step in this ongoing journey is to redefine your goals. While weight loss may have been your initial target, long-term success encompasses a broader perspective. Think about what health and wellness mean to you beyond the numbers on a scale. Perhaps it's about having more energy to play with your kids, reducing stress, improving your sleep, or feeling more confident in your skin. These are the goals that truly enrich your life and provide lasting motivation. Consider the habits that got you to this point. Which ones were most effective, and which ones could use some refinement? Maintaining success often involves solidifying these habits into your daily routine so they feel as automatic as brushing your teeth. This might include meal planning, regular exercise, mindful eating, and stress management techniques. These practices not only help maintain your weight but also contribute to your overall well-being. It's also important to keep learning and stay curious about nutrition and fitness. The field of health and wellness is ever-evolving, and staying informed can help you make educated choices. Experiment with new foods, try different workouts, and explore various methods of self-care.

This not only keeps things interesting but also allows you to discover what works best for your body and lifestyle. Another crucial aspect of long-term success is flexibility. Life is unpredictable, and rigid plans can easily fall apart when unexpected events occur. Being flexible means having the ability to adapt your routine without feeling like you've failed. Maybe it means swapping a gym session for a long walk with a friend or finding healthier options when dining out. Flexibility allows you to navigate the ups and downs of life while still prioritizing your health. Accountability is a powerful tool in maintaining long-term success. Whether it's a friend, family member, or health coach, having someone to share your journey with can provide support and encouragement. They can help you stay on track, celebrate your victories, and offer guidance when you encounter challenges. Even self-accountability tools, like keeping a journal or using a fitness app, can be effective in tracking your progress and maintaining focus. Your relationship with food also plays a significant role in sustaining long-term success. It's important to develop a mindset that views food as fuel and nourishment rather than a reward or punishment. Practice mindful eating by savoring each bite, recognizing hunger and fullness cues, and making conscious choices. This approach not only enhances your enjoyment of food but also helps prevent mindless eating that can derail your efforts. Finding balance is key. While maintaining a healthy lifestyle is important, it's equally vital to allow yourself some indulgences. Life is meant to be enjoyed, and occasional treats can be part of a balanced diet. The key is moderation, allowing yourself to enjoy without guilt and returning to your healthy habits afterward. This balance prevents feelings of deprivation and keeps you motivated to stay on track. Celebrating your successes, both big and small, is essential. Each milestone reached, whether it's maintaining your weight for another month or trying a new fitness class, is worth recognizing. These celebrations reinforce positive behaviors and remind you of how far you've come. They also provide motivation to keep moving forward, knowing that you are capable of achieving your goals. Visualize your future self and what a healthy lifestyle looks like for you in the long term. Envision how you want to feel, the activities you want to enjoy, and the life you want to lead. This visualization can be a powerful motivator, guiding your decisions and actions. It reminds you that your journey is not just about the present moment but also about creating a future that aligns with your values and aspirations. Embrace the journey as a lifelong commitment to health and happiness. Understand that there will be setbacks, but these are simply opportunities for growth and learning. Each challenge faced and overcome is a testament to your resilience and determination. With every step you take, you are building a foundation of health that will serve you for years to come. Finally, remember that you are not alone. Many have walked this path before you, and many will walk it after you. By sharing your journey and connecting with others, you contribute to a community of support and inspiration. Together, you can celebrate successes, share tips, and offer encouragement. This sense of community not only enriches your journey but also empowers you to stay committed to your goals.

4. Celebrating Milestones

Achieving any significant goal in life is a journey, not a single leap. Along this path, celebrating milestones becomes an essential practice that can sustain motivation and provide a sense of accomplishment. In the context of a weight loss journey or any health-related endeavor, recognizing these milestones is not merely about acknowledging progress; it's about affirming the hard work and dedication that goes into making lasting changes. Picture yourself climbing a mountain. The peak represents your ultimate goal, but the journey is made up of countless steps along the way. Each step taken is a small victory that brings you closer to the summit. Celebrating milestones along this path is like pausing at a scenic overlook to appreciate the view and recognize how far you've come. These moments of celebration are not distractions; they are integral to maintaining the momentum needed to reach the top. The first step in celebrating milestones is to identify what they mean to you. Milestones can be as varied and unique as the individuals who set them. For some, a milestone might be reaching a certain number on the scale, while for others, it might be fitting into a favorite pair of jeans or completing a challenging workout without fatigue. Milestones can also be non-scale victories, such as improved energy levels, better sleep, or a newfound sense of confidence. Recognizing and celebrating these achievements helps build a positive mindset and reinforces the behaviors that contribute to success. Celebrating milestones offers an opportunity for reflection. It allows you to look back at the journey so far, appreciating the challenges overcome and the lessons learned. This reflection can be a powerful motivator, reminding you of your strengths and resilience. It reinforces the idea that change is possible and that you are capable of achieving your goals. Reflecting on your progress can also help identify areas for further growth, offering insights that can guide your path forward. The act of celebrating should be meaningful and personal. It doesn't have to be grand or extravagant; rather, it should resonate with you and align with your values. Some may choose to celebrate with a special meal, a day of relaxation, or a new piece of workout gear. Others might find joy in sharing their success with loved ones, creating a sense of community and support. The key is to choose a form of celebration that brings you joy and satisfaction, reinforcing the positive emotions associated with your achievements. Celebrating milestones also serves as a reminder of why you started your journey in the first place. It reconnects you with your motivations and aspirations, reigniting the passion and commitment that fuel your progress. This renewed focus can be particularly valuable during times when motivation wanes or obstacles arise. By celebrating how far you've come, you reaffirm your dedication to reaching your ultimate goals. Moreover, celebrating milestones can have a ripple effect, inspiring others around you. Sharing your successes can motivate friends and family who may be on their own journeys. Your story becomes a testament to the power of perseverance and determination, demonstrating that positive change is achievable. This sense of inspiration not only benefits others but also reinforces your own commitment to maintaining progress. Incorporating celebrations into your journey can also help break the cycle of all-or-nothing thinking. It encourages you to focus on progress rather than perfection, acknowledging that every step forward is valuable, even if it's small. This mindset shift fosters a more compassionate and realistic approach to goal-setting, reducing the pressure to achieve perfection and allowing for greater flexibility and adaptability. It's important to recognize that the journey to achieving long-term goals is rarely linear. There will be setbacks, plateaus, and moments of doubt. Celebrating milestones provides a buffer against these challenges, offering encouragement and reminding you of your capability to overcome adversity. It builds resilience, helping you bounce back stronger and more determined than before. Setting future milestones can also be part of the celebration process. As you reach one goal, consider what the next step might be. Setting new, achievable milestones keeps the journey dynamic and engaging, providing fresh motivation to continue progressing. These future goals can be adjusted as needed, allowing for a flexible and personalized approach that adapts to your evolving needs and circumstances. Ultimately, celebrating milestones is about cultivating a positive relationship with yourself and your journey. It's about acknowledging your efforts, embracing your successes, and nurturing a mindset that values progress and growth. By celebrating each step forward, you create a journey that is not only about reaching a destination but about enjoying and appreciating the process itself.

MEASUREMENT CONVERSION TABLE

Volume Conversions

Volume (Liquid)	US Customary Units	Metric Units
1 teaspoon	1 tsp	5 milliliters (ml)
1 tablespoon	1 tbsp	15 milliliters
1 fluid ounce	1 fl oz	30 milliliters
1 cup	1 cup	240 milliliters
1 pint	1 pt	473 milliliters
1 quart	1 qt	946 milliliters
1 gallon	1 gal	3.785 liters

Weight Conversions

Weight	US Customary Units	Metric Units
1 ounce	1 oz	28 grams (g)
1 pound	1 lb	454 grams
1 kilogram	2.2 lbs	1000 grams (1 kg)

Length Conversions

Length	US Customary Units	Metric Units
1 inch	1 in	2.54 centimeters (cm)
1 foot	1 ft	30.48 centimeters

Metric Volume Conversions

Volume	Metric Units	US Customary Units
1 milliliter (ml)	1 ml	0.034 fluid ounce (fl oz)
100 milliliters	100 ml	3.4 fluid ounces
1 liter (L)	1 L	34 fluid ounces
		4.2 cups
		2.1 pints
		1.06 quarts
		0.26 gallon

Metric Weight Conversions

Weight	Metric Units	US Customary Units
1 gram (g)	1 g	0.035 ounces (oz)
100 grams	100 g	3.5 ounces
500 grams	500 g	1.1 pounds (lb)
1 kilogram (kg)	1 kg	2.2 pounds

Temperature Conversions

Temperature	Celsius (°C)	Fahrenheit (°F)
Freezing Point	0°C	32°F
Refrigerator	4°C	39°F
Room Temperature	20°C - 22°C	68°F - 72°F
Boiling Water	100°C	212°F